Doctor Nagler's Crash Diet

Lose 5-10 pounds your first week

Lose 10-20 pounds every month

Bill Nagler, M.D.
Diplomate, American Board of Weight Control Medicine
Diplomate, American Board of Psychiatry and Neurology

Gabrielle Nagler, M.A.

Diet Results
16311 Middlebelt
Livonia, Michigan 48154
800.511.9769 or 734.422.8040
www.dietresults.com

Doctor Nagler's Crash Diet

Lose 5-10 pounds your first week.
Lose 10-20 pounds every month.

For further information on mail-order sales, wholesale or retail discounts, distribution, translations, and foreign rights, please contact the publisher.

Diet Results
16311 Middlebelt
Livonia MI 48154
U.S.A.

Telephone 734-422-8040
Toll Free 800-511-9769
Fax 734-422-8588
www.dietresults.com

First Edition September 2001
10 9 8 7 6 5 4 3 2 1

ISBN 0-9715023-0-7
Printed in U.S.A.

Acknowledgements

Thank you to Donna, Kelly, Lisa, Mercy, Shannon, Shawn and Sue, for your hard work and support in the office. A double thank you to Sue and Shannon for your tireless proofreading. And a very special thank you to Todd for keeping it all together.

Books, tapes, video, computer programs and wallet-size diet cards by Bill Nagler, M.D. and Gabrielle Nagler, M.A.

Books:

Doctor Nagler's Crash Diet
The Cellulite Diet
Therapeutic Cuisine
The Dirty Half Dozen

Tapes:

Stay On Your Diet: Sweets Cravings
Stay On Your Diet: Starch Cravings
Stay On Your Diet: Motivation
Stop Smoking
Stop Drinking

Videos:

A Visit to the Diet Doctor

Computer Programs:

Hypnosis for Weight Loss
Hypnosis to Stop Smoking
Hypnosis to Stop Drinking
Hypnosis for Chronic Pain

Wallet-Size Diet Cards:

10-Days-10-Pounds-Off Program
Doctor Nagler's 500 Diet
No-Brainer Maintenance
Doctor Nagler's Formula Diet

Diet Results
16311 Middlebelt
Livonia, Michigan 48154
800-511-9769 or 734-422-8040
www.dietresults.com

Table of Contents

Doctor's Note 9

If You're In A Real Hurry 10

Introduction 11

Chapter 1
Dr. Nagler's Crash Diet 13
The Virtue of Weight Cycling
The Secret To Keeping Weight Off
Exercise and Weight Control
Stop Eating The Average American Diet
The Virtue Of Crash Diets
My Premium Crash Diets
How Long Can You Be On A Crash Diet?
Staying On Your Diet

Chapter 2
Ketosis: The Fat-Burning State 23
Ketogenic Diets
Ketosis
Counting Carbohydrates
Checking For Ketosis
What Makes You Fat
Lose Fat, Not Muscle
Metabolic Setpoint
How To Lower Your Setpoint
Step 1: Dr. Nagler's Crash Diet
Step 2: Exercise

Chapter 3
Crash Diet Instructions 31
If You're Not Hungry, Don't Eat
Drink At Least 128 Ounces Of Water A Day
Equal and SweetNLow Tablets Only

Constipation And The Apple Blitz
The Crash Diet Rules: The Short Version
The Crash Diet Rules: The Long Version
Helpful Hints
Frequently Asked Questions
Eating In Restaurants
Holidays
Ketogenic Lunch-On-The-Run

Chapter 4
Dr. Nagler's 10-Days-10-Pounds-Off Program 51
In A Nutshell: 10-Days-10-Pounds-Off
Original Phony Mayo Clinic Diet
Full Version: 10-Days-10-Pounds-Off
2 Tips To Make It Easier

Chapter 5
Dr. Nagler's 500 Diet 77
In A Nutshell: Dr. Nagler's 500 Diet
Full Version: Dr. Nagler's 500 Diet

Chapter 6
Other Options 97
Dr. Nagler's Very Low Fat Ketogenic Diet
Dr. Nagler's Ketogenic Crash
Dr. Nagler's Rotation Diet
Group I Rotations
Group II Rotations

Chapter 7
How To Stay On A Diet 115
The Myth Of Low Self Esteem
The Attitude Of The Thin
A Study On "Being Hungry"
Flooding
Implosion Therapy
Motivating Implosion

Table of Contents

Positive Implosion 1-12
Negative Implosion 1-12
Implosion Study

Chapter 8
Now That You've Lost The Weight 171
You Can't Go Back To Your Old Ways
Exercise
No-Brainer Maintenance Program
So What About Cheating?
Menu Suggestions

Chapter 9
A Visit To The Diet Doctor 178
What To Expect
Dr. Nagler's Formula Program
Prescription Medication
Diet-By-Mail
Implosion Tapes

About the Authors 191

Doctor's Note

Please don't follow my 10-Days-10-Pounds-Off Program or Dr. Nagler's 500 Diet, or any of the accelerated crash diet programs in this book, without the approval and supervision of your personal physician.

Make an appointment now for a medical check up. Remove one of the diet tear-out sheets in this book and give it to your doctor at the time of your visit. There are 3 copies of each diet in the book for this reason. The tear-out sheets for my 10-Days-10-Pounds-Off Program are on pages 71, 73 and 75. The tear-out sheets for Dr. Nagler's 500 Diet are on pages 91, 93 and 95.

If your doctor doesn't want you to go on my 10-Days-10-Pounds-Off Program or Dr. Nagler' 500 Diet, don't.

Bill Nagler, M.D.
October 2001

If You're In A Real Hurry

This book contains my 2 most popular crash diet programs, and many others.

Get your doctor's permission first, then go on either:

Dr. Nagler's 10-Days-10-Pounds-Off Program
(page 71)

OR

Dr. Nagler's 500 Diet
(page 91)

Call me any time for questions or support.

Bill Nagler, M.D.
Diet Results
16311 Middlebelt
Livonia, Michigan 48154

Telephone 734-422-8040
Toll Free 800-511-9769
Fax 734-422-8588
www.dietresults.com

Introduction

You've got to stop kidding yourself. You're probably not going to keep it off this time either. You never have before, why on earth are you going to now?

My Crash Diet is not the last diet you're ever going to go on, or the second to last. It's not going to change your eating habits forever or make you model-slim for eternity. It just ain't gonna happen.

What will happen, is that my Crash Diet will take a bunch of weight off you in a hurry. You can be down 5-10 pounds your first week, and drop 5 pounds every week after that.

My Crash Diet is about getting you to drop a quick 30 pounds for your high school reunion that's only two months away. Or helping you to shed a quick 20 pounds so you can fit into that slinky negligee you bought (a size too small) for your anniversary next month. Or finally making it possible for you to take off that stubborn 5 pounds in time for the family picture next week.

My Crash Diet is not forever, but for quick weight loss right now. Whether you follow my 10-Days-10-Pounds-Off Program (See Chapter 4) or Dr. Nagler's 500 (See Chapter 5), you will drop a bucket of weight in a hurry. But you won't keep it off. No one can promise you that.

Pay no attention to people who claim that they have a forever diet program for you. Like the man behind the curtain, they're just plain lying.

It's not that keeping weight off is impossible; it's just unlikely. The reality is that based on more than 20 years of practicing weight loss medicine, living in the diet trenches, I have found that most people are not willing to make the lifestyle changes and dietary sacrifices necessary to lose weight and keep it off for good. There are volumes of medical research to back me up on this.

Even so, I can help you to keep your weight off longer. If you follow my No-Brainer Maintenance Program (See Chapter 8) you will double the time you stay thin. My No-Brainer Maintenance Program is so easy. No one will ever know that you are on a maintenance program unless you tell them.

But, forget about maintenance for now. We'll talk about it later, after the reunion.

See your personal physician immediately. You should get medical approval before starting any weight loss program. Then go on either of my premium crash diets: Dr. Nagler's 10-Days-10-Pounds-Off Program (See Chapter 4) or Dr. Nagler's 500 Diet (See Chapter 5). You should be down 5-10 pounds your first week.

Chapter 1

Dr. Nagler's Crash Diet

I've been in the trenches fighting fat for twenty years now. During that time, I've treated more than 10,000 patients. Chances are, if you happened to live in the Detroit area any time during the past two decades, and you saw a diet doctor, you saw me.

From my experience, I can say with certainty that there is no magic bullet, potion or pill that will miraculously burn fat and keep it off forever. There is no magic. There is no little man behind the curtain. The emperor is naked indeed. It is unlikely that you have in your hands the perfect life-changing diet that will make you slim forever.

But what I can offer you is a way to safely take off a bucket of weight in a hurry, and keep it off, at least until the reunion or cruise or anniversary or whatever. And then soon after your landmark event, if you're like most people, you'll put back on every ounce you have lost. But don't worry, when you're ready to get back on the diet wagon, you'll take it off again.

The Virtue of Weight Cycling

Taking weight off and putting it back on again is not necessarily a bad thing. It's called weight cycling, and despite whatever garbage you may have read in a woman's magazine or in the tabloids, weight cycling or yo-yo dieting is actually good for you. Or more precisely, it's far better for you than staying fat.

Let's say you weigh 160 pounds, and over two months with me, you drop a quick 30. Believe me, it can happen. Even better results are possible. My current record is 29 pounds in one week. Last year Stephen came in weighing 293 pounds and one week later weighed in at 264.

But back to you. So you're down 30 pounds. You stay there for a while and then over the next 6 months you put every ounce back on again. Even so, you're actually far healthier having lost the weight and putting it back on, than not having lost the weight at all.

The reason is simple. Extra weight adds stress to your heart. Every pound of fat requires your heart to pump a mile of blood per day. So if you are down 30 pounds, that is 30 miles of blood per day that your heart no longer has to pump. And even when you gain back 5, 10 or 15 pounds, the heart is still not working as hard as it would if you had maintained your weight of 160. Losing the weight took the strain off your heart, at least for a while, which is what much of the health benefit of weight loss is in the first place. Losing weight, even temporarily, reduces your risk of heart disease, stroke and cancer, as well as relieves stress to the bones and joints, thereby decreasing symptoms of back pain and arthritis.

My program is designed to drop a bucket of weight in a hurry. I assume you're probably going to put it all back on again some time, but that doesn't worry me. Because while your weight is down, you're slimmer and healthier, which is at least a step in the right direction.

I repeat, if you truly want to lose weight and keep it off for good, the odds are against you, by 98%. However, if you are committed and disciplined, there is a chance. You could fall into the lucky 2% of people who have successfully maintained their weight loss.

The Secret To Keeping Weight Off

So what's the secret? How do the lucky 2% do it? How do they lose weight and keep it off for good?

The answer is so simple. Basically there are two cardinal rules that you must follow if you want to get down to your ideal weight and stay there:

(1) exercise for about 45 minutes a day 4-5 days a week, and

(2) stop eating the average American diet.

Exercise and Weight Control

Most people find it very hard to follow a regular exercise program. Although many belong to health and fitness clubs, most do not exercise on a regular basis. The pattern is one of fits and starts. How many times have you started an exercise regime, and found that after 3 months, you lost interest or just didn't have the time to get to the club, go for a run or whatever?

In my practice, the best predictor of whether or not a patient will start an exercise program and stick to it, is directly linked to whether that person is already following an exercise program at the time they first walk into my office.

According to studies conducted by exercise physiologist Paffenburger, long term exercise compliance is generally very low. His results show that less than 2% of the people who start an exercise program are going to still be exercising 2 years later. In fact, in the repeat of one of Paffenburger's studies in Beverly Hills, the only people who were still exercising at the end of 2 years were wealthy unemployed women. The researchers argued that it was the job of these women to stay thin for their husbands.

So, the odds are not good that once you

have lost weight, that you will keep it off with exercise. Unless of course, you fall into that small category of people who will actually follow a regular exercise program. According to Gunther and Gurin's classic long term study on weight loss, about 2% of people who lose weight, can keep it off for 2 years, the same 2% percent of people who exercise.

Stop Eating The Average American Diet

The other thing you have to do to lose weight for good is to stop eating garbage, meaning that you have to get off the average American diet.

Americans could learn a lot from the Japanese. The Japanese have the longest life expectancy on the planet. This is due to Western medical care, and an ultra low-fat diet of rice, fish, vegetables and seaweed. They hardly ever eat bread, butter, cheese, dairy products or dessert.

I try to eat this way myself and highly recommend it. The Japanese diet is not only healthy but terrific for keeping weight under control.

Unfortunately, the Japanese diet is hard to follow. Most Americans can't imagine giving up dairy products and bread. Plus the thought of seaweed is most unappealing. And if you eat out a lot, as most Americans do (about 3-4 times a week), controlling your fat intake can be a problem. Most restaurants cook with way too much butter and oil. And portions are generally too large.

To let the reality of this sink in, next time you go to a restaurant, sit at a table with a clear view of the kitchen. Just watch how much oil, butter and sauce is added to "light" or "low-fat" dishes. You will be amazed.

So, what can you do to stay thin? I'll tell you what I do.

I'm fifty, five feet nine inches, and weigh 150 pounds. To maintain my weight, I do just what you probably won't. I sweat my brains out in the basement, for forty-five minutes, five times a week on my Schwinn elliptical machine, next to Gabrielle (my wife) sweating it out on the treadmill. And even worse, more often than not, I live on rice, fish, vegetables and seaweed.

But I don't expect you or any of my patients to exercise and eat the way I do. Because if you are like most people, the idea of committing to a regular exercise program and a radical change in diet is just plain unappealing. For some of you, practicality is the issue. In any case, I have found that its always something.

The reality is, after you lose weight on my program, you are more likely than not, going to slowly put it all back on again. The odds are that you are going to eventually regain every ounce you have lost, unless you get religion (exercise) and dramatically (impossibly?) change your dietary habits. You're going to have to make an all-out, radical lifestyle change to keep it off for good - not very likely, at least not for most people.

You may think that I am being negative, but I prefer to call it realistic. My goal is not to depress you, but to offer you reasonable expectations and to lay out appropriate strategies for dealing with the battle of the bulge. Don't feel defeated. There is a way out. And you've known it all along.

The Virtue Of Crash Diets

You know from experience that even if you lose a bucket of weight, it is very likely that at some point in time, you're going to gain every ounce back. And you probably think that is a very bad thing. That's where I disagree.

The fact that you can successfully lose a bucket of weight is a good thing. If you can do it once, you can do it twice or three times. And unless you want to radically change your lifestyle, the only way you can keep weight off is to go on and off diets. Just make sure that those diets are safe, protein sufficient and work. And mine are all those things. Like my patients, you can lose weight on my crash diet, keep it off for a while, and then go back on and lose the weight again. And again, and again.

To keep your weight off as long as possible, I strongly suggest you follow my No-Brainer Maintenance Program (See Chapter 8). Chances are, being human and not exercising, your weight will gradually creep on again. But my No-Brainer Maintenance Diet can double the time you stay thin, based on the experience of thousands of my patients.

My Premium Crash Diets: The 10-Days-10-Pounds-Off Program and Dr. Nagler's 500 Diet

The fastest and most popular crash diet programs I use on 95% of my patients are the 10-Days-10-Pounds-Off and the 500 Diet. These diets are designed to take off 5-10 pounds your first week, and about 5 pounds every week thereafter. You shouldn't feel hungry. And no one will ever know you are on a diet unless you tell them.

How Long Can You Be On A Crash Diet?

Most of my patients stay on my programs anywhere from 3 days (to drop a quick 5 pounds) to 3-4 weeks (to drop a quick 15-20 pounds). In general, I don't recommend crash dieting for much more than 1-2 months at a time, even with medical supervision. Dieting is hard, hard work, and you need to give yourself a break. Take a week or two off after a month of dieting if you still have weight you want to lose, and follow my No-Brainer Maintenance program.

After a couple of weeks on No-Brainer, go back to my 10-Days-10-Pounds-Off Program, Dr. Nagler's 500 Diet or any of my other crash diet programs.

So, I'm assuming that you want to drop a quick 10-40 pounds, and that you have your personal physician's blessing and approval at this point.

The best way to start is to jump in with both feet and follow either my 10-Days-10-Pounds-Off Program or Dr. Nagler's 500 Diet, outlined in the Chapters 4 and 5. You can follow either program from 3 days (to drop a quick 5 pounds) to 1-2 months (to drop 20-40 pounds).

Staying On Your Diet

After a few days on either my 10-Days-10-Pounds-Off Program or Dr. Nagler's 500 Diet, you may need some help to stay motivated (as you do on all diets; you're allowed to be human).

Half of losing weight is making a decision or a commitment to stay on your diet. And it's particularly easy to fall off the wagon. Sara Lee and

McDonald's aren't planning to go out of business, so temptation is always going to be there for you. It's awfully hard to near impossible to lose weight if you're constantly cheating.

Based on research I conducted at the University of Michigan and a paper I wrote for Psychological Reports, I have discovered a way to keep you from falling off every diet you go on. I call it Implosion Therapy, which is discussed in great detail in Chapter 7 - How To Stay On A Diet. With the help of my Implosion Therapy, you can keep on dieting until you have reached your goal.

Chapter 2

Ketosis: The Fat-Burning State

Ketogenic Diets

In my 20 years of clinical experience, I have found Ketogenic Diets to be the most effective for weight loss. Ketogenic Diets are very low in carbohydrate and very high in protein.

Low carbohydrate diets have been around for a long time. In 1863, William Banting published the world's first ketogenic quick weight loss diet, his "Letter on Corpulence". The diet was reborn in the 1950's as Dr. Tallman's Calories Don't Count, in the 1960's as Dr. Stillman's Quick Weight Loss Diet, in the 1970's as Dr. Atkin's Diet Revolution, in the 1980's as Dr. Linn's Last Chance Diet, and in the 1990's as Barry Sear's Zone Diet.

Ketogenic Diets entered mainstream medicine in the 1950's through the work and clinical experience of the late Dr. A.T.W. Simeons. Simeons believed that ketogenic diets actually help your body break down fat faster than normal. His methods and techniques have been modified over the years, and are now being used by physicians across the country on thousands of patients every day.

Ketosis

Ketosis is the process of dissolving fat, breaking it down into ketones which are released through the breath and the urine. In ketosis, you are using protein for body fuel instead of sugar. The way to do this is to eat protein and to practically eliminate carbohydrates (starches and sweets) from your diet.

Using sugar or carbohydrates for fuel elevates insulin levels. Insulin converts excess carbohydrates into fat. So if you have a tendency to eat too many carbohydrates, guess what happens. You got it. You store more fat which makes you gain weight.

As you decrease carbohydrates in your diet, insulin levels drop. On a low carbohydrate or ketogenic diet, insulin levels are low enough so that fat is burned and no longer stored.

Counting Carbohydrates

To be in ketosis, your carbohydrate intake should be between 10 and 20 grams a day. There are carbohydrate counter books available that give you the exact number of carbohydrates contained in most foods. In general, lean meat, chicken, fish, and some cheeses have a zero carbohydrate count.

Grains, either whole or processed, have a very high carbohydrate count. Vegetables vary in their carbohydrate count. Sweet vegetables like carrots and corn have a high carbohydrate count whereas watery, leafy vegetables like lettuce and spinach have a very low carbohydrate value. Most fruits contain a lot of carbohydrates. Some are worse than others. For example, grapes are high, and strawberries are low.

The more grams of carbohydrates your body takes in, the slower your weight loss. If you're not careful and your carbohydrates go above 20 grams per day, you are out of ketosis and not in an efficient fat-burning, weight loss state.

My 10-Days-10-Pounds-Off and 500 Diets make dieting simpler and weight loss quicker by basically cutting out foods that are high in carbohydrates. Counting carbohydrates is not necessary. Your food choices are simple and straightforward.

Being on a ketogenic diet gives you a metabolic advantage. Studies have shown that calorie-for-calorie, you will lose weight much faster on a ketogenic diet than any other type of weight loss program.

Checking For Ketosis

To make sure you are in a fat-burning state, you must check your urine daily for ketosis. The best way to do this is with Ketostix (available in my office or any drugstore). Dip the colored end of a Ketostix strip in a fresh urine specimen or pass it through a stream of urine. After 15 seconds compare the color of the end of your strip with the color chart on the side of your Ketostix bottle.

If your strip is medium pink, you are in small or moderate ketosis, which is where you want to be. If the strip shows pale pink or beige, you are not in ketosis. At this point, you should eliminate all carbohydrates from your diet. If the strip shows medium or dark purple, you are dehydrated and must drink more water.

Make sure to buy Ketostix that test for urine ketones only. Also check the expiration date of your Ketostix before using them.

What Makes You Fat

There are many factors than cause weight gain. The most common is eating too much. Medical causes of obesity are rare, but include inherited genetic characteristics, glandular disorders of the thyroid, pituitary, adrenal and sex glands, and metabolic disorders such as diabetes or hypoglycemia.

Certain medications can contribute to weight gain, such as cortisone, certain antidepressants and birth control pills. Psychological factors may also play a role.

Regardless of the cause, obesity can be treated effectively with a Ketogenic Diet. Obesity is a problem that must be treated properly and controlled for the rest of one's life.

Lose Fat, Not Muscle

The weight loss from a Ketogenic Diet is primarily of fat tissue that has been stored in the abdomen, waist, hips and thighs. Non-ketogenic diets, on the other hand, tend to be protein deficient and can therefore result in a loss of normal essential muscle tissue. The muscle loss tends to create a pale, shallow appearance of the face and neck, and can produce symptoms of malnutrition such as hunger, fatigue, dizziness, lightheadedness, dehydration, lethargy, irritability and mild depression. Dieters on non-ketogenic diets often complain of losing weight from the wrong areas of their body.

Metabolic Setpoint

A ketogenic diet can also help to lower your Metabolic Setpoint. Your Metabolic Setpoint is the weight your body is genetically programmed to weigh.

Let's say you weigh 160 pounds, and you diet your way down to 130 pounds. Although you are 30 pounds lighter than when you started your diet, you still experience the hunger you had at 160 pounds.

So any time your will-power fades, or someone gives you a dirty look, or you are stressed, you eat and eat, until you eventually get right back up to 160 pounds.

The reason that you regain the weight is that 160 pounds is your metabolic setpoint. Your metabolic setpoint is genetically predetermined. It is amount of weight that your body is physiologically programmed to weigh.

Look at your parents and siblings. You likely have a similar build to at least one of your family members. Most people in the same family are shaped the same way. They all carry about the same weight for their height and bone-structure proportionally. This is genetically determined and referred to as your setpoint. Your setpoint controls how hungry you are, how much you want to eat, and how much your body wants to weigh.

Even so, there is no reason to be discouraged, there are ways to lower your setpoint.

How To Lower Your Setpoint

There are two ways of lowering your setpoint in order to lose weight. You can go on a special ketogenic diet or you can exercise. I recommend both.

Step 1: Dr. Nagler's Crash Diet

My premium crash diets, The 10-Days-10-Pounds-Off Program and Dr. Nagler's 500 Diet are ketogenic, low carbohydrate diets which help to lower your insulin levels to such a degree that you can lower your setpoint. You eat less and experience less hunger, and as a result lower your setpoint by decreasing the percentage of fat that your body is carrying. On average, you can lose 5-10 pounds the first week and 10-20 pounds a month.

Step 2: Exercise

The more you exercise, the more calories you burn, of course. And the more calories you burn, the faster you lose weight. But in terms of resetting your setpoint, exercise is almost useless, unless you exercise at least five days a week, forty-five minutes a day. You need at least this much regular exercise in order to significantly drop your setpoint, and keep it down.

As most people don't have the time or inclination for this much physical activity, I don't recommend exercise for lowering setpoint. However, I do recommend exercise to burn calories.

For every mile you run or walk, you burn about a hundred calories. Remember, it doesn't matter how quickly you cover the mile in terms of caloric consumption. Running a mile burns the same number of calories as walking a mile. The distance covered is the key.

Exercise will make you burn more calories, and lose weight faster. The more you exercise, the better you will feel. And you'll live longer, too. But exercise is only effective for resetting setpoint if you can do it five days a week, forty-five minutes a day.

Exercise as much as you can. Just make sure to get your personal physician's approval first, especially if you are morbidly obese or have heart problems.

Chapter 3

Crash Diet Instructions

If You're Not Hungry, Don't Eat

The most important thing you have to do to lose weight as rapidly as possible on my 10-Days-10-Pounds-Off Program or Dr. Nagler's 500 Diet is:

If you're not hungry, don't eat. I'll say it again. If you're not hungry, don't eat.

Don't eat breakfast or anything at all if you're not hungry. The less you eat, the faster you will lose on either of these rapid crash diets.

It's as simple as that. If you're not hungry, don't eat. There's no magic. The less you eat, the faster you will lose weight. After 2-3 days you'll be in the fat-burning state of ketosis (See Chapter 2) on either diet, so you should not be particularly hungry, so not eating will be a lot easier than it sounds.

You don't have to eat all the food or all the meals on either program. Once again: the less you eat, the faster you will lose weight and inches. Got it?

Drink At Least 128 Ounces Of Water A Day

The second most important thing you have to do on both programs, is to drink your water. You have to, have to, have to drink at least 128 ounces of water a day. 150 or 200 ounces of water a day is even better. You have to drink your water to lose weight and feel at your best on these very rapid crash diet programs. You will be in ketosis (See Chapter 2), so you really need to push fluids to flush out your fat as you experience very speedy weight loss.

Remember on ketogenic diets (See Chapter 2) like the 10-Days-10-Pounds-Off Program and Dr. Nagler's 500 Diet, you are expelling a lot of fat through the urine, so drinking a lot of water is absolutely imperative. You do not want to get dehydrated nor do you want to stress your kidneys.

Once you are in ketosis, the ketogenic state should help block your appetite, accelerate fat burning, and keep your energy up.

You can't drink too much water or fluid on this program. The more you drink the better you will do, and the better you will feel. You need at least a gallon (128 ounces) of fluid a day to flush out the fat you are burning on this very rapid quick weight loss crash diet program.

You will feel at your best if you can drink at least your weight in ounces of water. For example, if your current weight is 150 pounds, you should try to drink at least 150 ounces of water a day on my crash diet programs. If you weigh 250 pounds and want to lose weight, you need to try to drink at least 250 ounces of water a day. I'm not kidding. It's almost impossible to drink too much water. Check with your doctor who is supervising you, if you don't believe me.

Equal And SweetNLow Tablets Only (No Packets), No Flavored Coffee, No Creamer

You may add Equal or SweetNLow tablets to your coffee or tea if you need a sweetener. But NO Equal or SweetNLow packets. The packets contain more carbohydrate than the tablets, and can get you into trouble by knocking you out of ketosis and triggering feelings of hunger. To get into the quick fat-burning state of ketosis, you will be drastically limiting your carbohydrate intake.

Absolutely no flavored coffees, coffee creamers, coffee whitener or cappuccino. The carbohydrate content is way too high for my crash diets. The little extra carbohydrate can quickly knock you out of ketosis, and stop you from losing weight.

You may only have diet drinks that are 0-calorie AND 0-carbohydrate. That means that you can drink all the canned or bottled diet soda (Diet Coke, Diet Seven-Up, Diet Doctor Pepper, etc.) you can pour down. No other diet drinks are allowed on my 10-Days-10-Pounds-Off Program or Dr. Nagler's 500 Diet.

Any sweetener or drink with more than a 0-calorie and 0-carbohydrate count is off limits. That includes sweeteners or drinks labeled as having less than one gram of carbohydrate per serving. The reason for this restriction is due to a loophole in the U.S. labeling law which allows manufacturers not to list one 1/2 gram of carbohydrate per serving. This means that something labeled as having one gram of carbohydrate may in fact have 1.5 grams of carbohydrate, or possibly more.

And given that I am asking you to drink a lot of fluids, those 1/2 grams of carbohydrates can really add up. So stay away from powdered sweeteners and powdered diet drinks. Your carbohydrate intake can rapidly get out of control.

Constipation And The Apple Blitz

You will more likely than not experience very mild constipation on either my 10-Days-10-Pounds-Off or 500 Diet Program. Very little is going in, so very little is coming out. Forgetdaboudid.

If the constipation is totally driving you nuts on either program, take a day off and with your doctor's permission go on my Apple Blitz. On the Apple Blitz you eat 6 apples a day, and that's it. You can't have anything else, other than your 128 ounces of water.

The 6 apples will cause a little diarrhea and clean you out. Then go right back on my 10-Days-10-Pounds-Off Program or Dr. Nagler's 500 Diet.

If constipation is a real problem for you, you can go on the Apple Blitz once a week. If you are chronically constipated, you might want to clean yourself out before starting my 10-Days-10-Pounds-Off Program or Dr. Nagler's 500 Diet. The best way to do this is to go on my Apple Blitz for 1 day, and then start your diet.

The Crash Diet Rules: The Short Version

These rules are cast in stone, and apply to either my 10-Days-10-Pounds-Off Program or Dr. Nagler's 500 Diet, whichever program you decide to go on. If you don't follow my Crash Diet Rules, you won't lose weight as quickly and feel as well as you should.

1 - NO alcoholic beverages or coffee creamer/whitener.

2 - NO lozenges, cough drops, candy, ANY gum or breath mints.

3 - Use ONLY Breath Asure or Binaca spray for your breath.

4 - Use SweetNLow or Equal TABLETS only (NO powdered packets), except you may use 1 powdered packet on your half grapefruit if you want it sweeter.

5 - You must drink at least 4 quarts (128 ounces) of water a day.

The Crash Diet Rules: The Long Version

You have to follow these rules exactly, if you want to lose 5-10 pounds your first week on my programs, and 4-5 pounds every week thereafter. You CANNOT cheat or deviate from these guidelines at all. You also need to carefully follow my instructions to feel at your best on my very rapid crash diets.

(1) Drink at least a gallon (128 ounces) of water or noncaloric fluid a day.

This means you must drink about twelve 10-ounce glasses of water (or noncaloric fluid) a day. Drinking 150-200 ounces a day is even better. You need this much fluid to flush out your fat, and keep your kidneys healthy.

Water is the healthiest thing to drink, but coffee, tea, Diet Coke, and diet soda are fine. You don't have to drink water at all if you hate it (although you'll find once you get into the habit of drinking a lot of water, you'll learn to love it). But you must drink at least 128 ounces of noncaloric fluid a day, or you won't lose weight and stay healthy.

Once you are in ketosis, you can drink Diet Snapple or Crystal Lite - but only if you check your urine with Ketostix (See (3)) every time you urinate. If you can remain in ketosis drinking Diet Snapple and Crystal Lite, drink them. If not, throw them out. Absolutely NO regular pop or sugared drinks!

(2) Get into ketosis.

The best way to get into ketosis quickly and speed up your weight loss, is to eat only the MEAT list for 2-3 days on any of my programs. If you are very hungry, you may have a third serving of MEAT while you are getting into ketosis, but only if you do not have anything else. NO fruit, vegetables, or salads - nothing else until you are in ketosis, then follow the crash diets exactly as written.

Absolutely NO cheating. You can't cheat at all, if you want to get into ketosis to speed up your weight loss.

Rule (2) applies to all my crash diets except for the 10-Days-10-Pounds-Off Program which requires that you eat a 1/2 grapefruit before eating anything else.

(3) Use Ketostix to check whether you are in ketosis.

When you are in ketosis, you are burning fat at a very high rate. To check if you are in ketosis, use Ketostix. Dip the colored end of a Ketostix strip in a fresh urine specimen or pass it through a stream of urine. After 15 seconds compare the color of the end of your strip with the color chart on the side of your Ketostix bottle.

If your strip is medium pink, you are in small or moderate ketosis, which is where you want to be. If the strip shows pale pink or beige, you are not in ketosis. At this point, you should eliminate all carbohydrates from your diet (eat only protein). If the strip shows medium or dark purple, you are dehydrated and must drink more water.

Check your urine with Ketostix every time you urinate. If you are not in ketosis, stop cheating and get into ketosis in order to lose weight!

Ketostix can be purchased at my office, either directly or through the mail, or at any drugstore.

(4) No breath mints or gum are allowed until you are in ketosis.

Once you are in ketosis, you can chew sugarless gum and use sugarless breath mints, but only if you check your urine with Ketostix and can remain in ketosis after using them. For bad breath it's best to take 3 Breath Asure every 2-3 hours. Breath Asure is readily available and can also be purchased at my office either directly or through the mail.

(5) You CANNOT switch back and forth between my 10-Days-10-Pounds-Off Program and Dr. Nagler's 500 Diet every few days and expect to lose weight.

You must stay on either my 10-Days-10-Pounds-Off Program or Dr. Nagler's 500 Diet for at least a week before switching. NEVER combine the two diets.

This way, you should drop 5-10 pounds your first week, and 4-5 pounds every week thereafter.

(6) Finally, unless your doctor says otherwise, don't stay on my 10-Days-10-Pounds-Off Program or Dr. Nagler's 500 Diet for more than 2 months.

After every 20-30 pounds you lose, take a week or two off and go on my No-Brainer Maintenance Program. Give your body a break from rapid weight loss and fat burning. (See Chapter 8).

And remember, please don't go on any of my programs without medical supervision.

Helpful Hints

(1) Follow your diet

Eat foods from your food list only. Follow all of my instructions exactly. If at any time you are not hungry, don't eat. The less you eat, the faster you will lose weight. You do not have to finish everything on your plate, or eat three meals a day. If a food is not mentioned, you can't have it.

(2) Drink water

Drink at least 128 ounces of water a day. In addition to that, you may have coffee, tea, sparkling water and diet sodas. If you get hungry, drink a glass of noncaloric liquid before you even think of eating anything. You may find that your hunger fades.

(3) Avoid fat and sugar

Try to completely eliminate all butter, margarine, fat, and oil from your diet. Avoid sugar and honey like the plague. Read labels carefully when you go shopping to avoid unwanted sugar (carbohydrate) and fat.

(4) Exercise

Exercise is highly recommended for weight loss. Exercise 30-45 minutes a day, 5 days a week.

Frequently Asked Questions

(1) Don't I need to eat something, to keep my metabolism burning?

Absolutely not. Your body metabolism is always burning whether you eat or not. It does not significantly slow down or speed up throughout the day (unless you are exercising which gives your metabolism a bit of a push).

(2) I feel lightheaded. What's going on?

Drink more water. Lightheadedness is a normal side effect of dieting. Drink at least 128 ounces of water a day. Change position slowly, and your lightheadedness should go away.

(3) I'm craving sweets. What should I do?

If you have sweet cravings, stop all chicken, turkey, eggs, EggBeaters and cottage cheese for two or three days. Your sweet cravings should go away. Poultry and dairy products are loaded with hormones that can make you crave sweets.

(4) What can I do about my dry mouth?

Drink more water! If you are drinking your 128 ounces of water a day, dry mouth should not be a problem. If you are drinking at least a gallon of water a day and your mouth is still dry, take 500mg-1500mg of Evening Primrose capsules, one to three times a day.

(5) What can I do about my bad breath?

Try Breath Asure, three capsules every three or four hours. Drink eight to twelve ounces of water each time you take the capsules, and your breath will be fine. Remember to stay away from sugarless gum and breath mints, which kick you out of ketosis (See Chapter 2) and stop you from losing weight.

(6) Why do I have to drink so much water?

You need to drink at least 128 ounces of water a day (in addition to all the coffee, tea and diet pop you want) in order to flush out all the fat you are burning on my crash diets and avoid damage to your kidneys.

(7) Can I drink diet pop instead of water?

Yes, if you can't stand water. But you must drink at least 128 ounces a day.

(8) What can I eat for breakfast?

Before you even think about eating, drink at least a quart of noncaloric fluid, preferably water. If you are still hungry, then eat from your food list. Eat only from your food list, and eat as little as possible.

(9) What can I do to lose weight faster?

If you're not hungry, don't eat! Really pay attention to whether you are hungry or not. Avoid recreational eating or grazing. Unless you are truly hungry, don't eat. You can go for days without eating. But keep drinking your water.

(10) I'm not in ketosis. What's wrong?

You're taking in too many carbohydrates. Only eat from your MEAT list. Stop all fruits and vegetables. Make sure you are drinking your water. You should be in ketosis in 1-2 days.

(11) I can't sleep. Is something wrong?

Stop all caffeine (no Diet Coke, coffee or tea). Make sure that you are drinking at least 128 ounces of water a day. And get some exercise.

(12) Will eating so much protein raise my cholesterol?

Serum cholesterol is determined more by the fat stored in your body than by the fat in your diet. So if you lose weight, you lose stored fat which helps lower your cholesterol.

However, when you first start a high protein diet, your cholesterol will rise a bit. But as you begin to lose weight your cholesterol will fall.

(13) What can I eat in restaurants?

Anything that used to walk, swim, fly, run, or crawl, cooked without butter, margarine or oil. Order fish dry, and put lemon on it. Have two or three shrimp cocktails. Order an omelette made with EggBeaters or with a combination of four whites and one yolk. Have a steamed or broiled lobster. Have a hamburger without a bun or a scoop of tuna made with very little or preferably no mayonnaise.

Eating in Restaurants

Almost a third of your meals are eaten away from home today. So you need to know how to eat in restaurants while on a special diet, without feeling deprived. You shouldn't feel like you are being tortured, just because you are dining out. You are paying good money, for a good time.

All you have to do is ask for what you want. Ask for your food prepared dry, without butter, margarine or oil. Ask for your food broiled, baked, steamed or poached. Ask for sauces or dressings on the side. Or better yet, ask for low-fat or low-carbohydrate sauces or dressings. Ask for mustard, lemon juice, horseradish or hot sauce to add some flavor.

If you order something broiled, and it comes to you fried, send it back. If you order something dry, and it comes drenched in butter, send it back. If you ask for your salad with the dressing on the side, and it comes to you dressed, send it back.

Restaurants provide a service - cooking. And you're paying quite a bit for this service. So, have it your way. Be polite. But be firm. That way you'll get exactly what you want.

Holidays

Another big problem is holiday eating. But it doesn't have to be. Think about it. There are no calories in Christmas, Easter or Thanksgiving. There are no calories in your birthday, anniversary or graduation.

So, why do you put on weight at these times? The reason is simple. You increase your intake of fat. You eat too much cake or too many chips. You constantly have your hands in the candy bowl. You pile on the gravy and just have to have a second helping of Grandma's potatoes. You go to parties and eat when you aren't hungry.

As you increase your intake of fat, you want to eat more of everything else. The increase of fat calories raises your setpoint (See Chapter 2) and triggers feeding frenzy. So you eat, and eat, and eat. Your setpoint goes up and you gain weight.

So avoid putting on holiday pounds by watching your intake of fat. Keep your portions small. You can still enjoy holiday goodies with your friends and family. Just make the right choices. Choose one dessert instead of two or three, and don't eat the whole thing. Just take a bite or two. There's no rule that says that you have to lick your plate clean. And there is no need to try everything. You know what most of it tastes like anyway.

And limit your intake of alcohol. Alcohol stimulates the appetite and is also high in calories. I consider it the Great Enabler as far as dieting is concerned. But during the holidays, it is hard to abstain. My advice is:

(1) Have one drink or one dessert, not both.

(2) Whether you decide to have one drink or one dessert, have exactly what you want. For example, if you want white wine, don't settle for red. If you want chocolate ice cream, don't settle for vanilla. That way you'll be satisfied with less of whatever of you chose. As the saying goes, "You can never get enough of what you really don't want."

During the holidays, eat as little as possible. The less you eat, the less likely you will gain weight.

Ketogenic Lunch-On-The-Run

If you're out for lunch or dinner, and you just have to eat something, eating the foods on this list will keep you in ketosis. You're better off staying on my 10-Days-10-Pounds-Off or my 500 Diet, but this list is your fallback.

Quiche or pizza - no crust

Fajita - no tortilla, no guacamole, no sour cream

Roll-up sandwich - made with lettuce, not bread

Kabob - beef or chicken, no rice

Egg white or EggBeaters omelette

Salad - Cobb, Greek, Chef, Grilled Chicken, use low-fat or fat-free dressing

Shrimp cocktail

Fish - poached, steamed, broiled, grilled, cooked with no fat

Shellfish - poached, steamed, broiled, grilled, cooked with no fat

String cheese - low-fat or fat-free

Beef jerky - no brown sugar

Hot dog or Vienna sausage - no bun

Crash Diet Instructions

Tuna - made with lemon juice or fat-free mayonnaise

Arby's roast beef - no bun

Burger King - hamburger/broiled chicken, no bun, salad with low-fat dressing

Wendy's - hamburger/broiled chicken, no bun, salad with low-fat dressing

McDonald's - hamburger/broiled chicken, no bun, salad with low-fat dressing

Boston Chicken - chicken no skin

Chapter 4

Dr. Nagler's 10-Days-10-Pounds-Off Program

For those of you who want to cut to the chase and start losing weight in a hurry, here's the quick and dirty version of my 10-Days-10-Pounds-Off Program.

Full background and support information follows, but for those of you who want to start losing weight now, here's the program for you.

In a Nutshell: 10-Days-10-Pounds-Off

Most people can lose up to 10 pounds in 10 days on this program.

Follow my instructions exactly. If you're not hungry, don't eat.

Breakfast

1/2 Grapefruit

Coffee or Tea

Lunch

1/2 Grapefruit

Salad (up to 1 cup)

Bacos & EggBeaters (4 ounces EggBeaters with 1 tablespoon Bacos)
OR
Egg White Omelette (1 yolk and 4 whites)

Coffee or Tea

Dinner

1/2 Grapefruit

Salad (up to 1 cup)

Vegetable (up to 1 cup)

Meat (up to 8 ounces)

Coffee or Tea

Grapefruit

You must eat a 1/2 grapefruit before any meal. You don't have to eat all the food or meals on the list, but you must have the 1/2 grapefruit before eating anything else. If you are hungry in between meals, you may have a 1/2 grapefruit as a snack. No more than 3 whole grapefruit a day.

Add 1 Equal or SweetNLow packet to your grapefruit if you want it sweeter, but only use Equal or SweetNLow tablets for drinks.

Salad

Both lunch and dinner SALADS have a maximum total volume of 1 cup. SALAD consists only of the following vegetables in any combination: lettuce, cucumbers, mushrooms, onions, radishes and sprouts. You may use up to 2 tablespoons of a low-fat, low-carbohydrate dressing on your salad. That means no more than 3 grams of fat and no more than 3 grams of carbohydrate per single serving of dressing.

Vegetables

You may have up to 1 cup of only one of the following dinner VEGETABLES per day:

asparagus, broccoli, Brussels sprouts, cauliflower, mushrooms, sauerkraut, spinach, string beans.

Meat

You may have up to 8 ounces of only one of the following dinner MEATS per day:

chicken, clams, crab, fish (any), lobster, mussels, sardines, scallops, shrimp, tuna, turkey, veal.

No oil, no butter, no margarine, no breading on anything. Lemon juice, mustard and vinegar are okay.

No alcohol, no coffee creamer. No lozenges, no gum, no mints. Use Breath Asure capsules or Binaca spray instead.

Drink a minimum of 128 ounces (4 quarts) of water a day, 150 ounces is better. Don't eat anything else. If you're going out, bring grapefruit. No substitutions! No cheating! You'll melt!

So. That's my diet. Get your personal physician's permission, and you can start losing weight today. Now, for those of you who want the inside scoop, here's the background on the program.

Original Phony Mayo Clinic Diet

Dr. Nagler's 10-Days-10-Pounds-Off Program is an updated, safe, version of the Mayo Clinic Diet, the most popular diet in the country in the early 1970's.

The Mayo Clinic over the years has repeatedly disavowed any knowledge, connection or affiliation with this program, which first became popular when it was circulated around the offices of America on Xerox memos. This was well before the days of fax machines.

The Original Phony Mayo Clinic Diet had a number of strange and idiotic requirements. Even so, some people did manage to drop the promised 10 pounds in a week. The weight dropped was mostly water, given that the calorie count was so high. And as fast as the weight came off, it piled back on as soon as the dieters went back to normal eating.

You've got to promise not to even think about going on or trying the Original Phony Mayo Clinic Diet, but for the sake of history (and a little comic relief), I'm including it. Once again, the diet is not affiliated in any way with the prestigious Mayo Clinic in Rochester, Minnesota.

Okay. So here's the Original Phony Mayo Clinic Diet along with my running commentary. Don't even think about going on this program. It is totally nuts.

Don't Eat This Breakfast

1/2 Grapefruit

12 Eggs and 12 strips of Bacon

Coffee or tea (just 1 cup)

I'm not kidding here. On the Original Phony Mayo Clinic Diet, you could have as many eggs as you wanted, up to a dozen, with up to a dozen strips of bacon. The requirement was that you had to eat at least 1 egg and 1 strip of bacon, whether you were hungry or not. In addition, for every egg you ate, you had to have 1 strip of bacon, whether you wanted it or not. The eggs could be cooked in loads of butter, or any way you wanted.

Doing the numbers, this means that on the Original Phony Mayo Clinic Diet, you could have up to 2160 calories in bacon and eggs alone just for breakfast. Adding 50 calories for your grapefruit half, you're up to more than 2200 calories before you start your day, whether you're hungry or not! You were also limited to just one cup of coffee or tea. The diet was quite firm on this point, no more than one cup of coffee or tea.

Don't Eat This Lunch

1/2 Grapefruit

Salad with Olive Oil, quantity unlimited

Meat with butter, quantity unlimited

Coffee or tea (just 1 cup)

The salad had to be topped with olive oil and vinegar (as much as you wanted!), and you could have as much meat as you could eat, topped with butter. Doing the numbers here again, you've got at least 400 calories for a large salad topped with olive oil, and at least another 1000 calories for the meat, assuming you had a 12 ounce steak. So, counting the grapefruit half, you're at almost 1500 calories for lunch, not counting your 2200 calorie breakfast. The only thing you were limited on was coffee or tea. You could only have one cup. (Guess where the weight loss on this program came from - you're right, dehydration!)

Don't Eat This Dinner

1/2 Grapefruit

Salad with Olive Oil, quantity unlimited

Meat with butter, quantity unlimited

Vegetable with butter, quantity unlimited

Coffee or tea (just 1 cup)

You could eat as much low carbohydrate vegetable as you wanted, drained of all liquid before serving. Draining the liquid cut the carbohydrates down. Then you could top your vegetable with as much butter as you wanted.

The addition of a generously buttered vegetable added another 400 calories to your 1500 calorie lunch, bringing dinner alone up to 1900 calories, more than the break-even caloric point for the average American woman. Coffee and tea were still limited to just one cup.

Doing the numbers, you could easily have eaten in excess of 5000 calories a day on this program. All the weight loss on the Original Phony Mayo Clinic Diet was due to severe dehydration, created by restricting fluid intake to 3 cups of coffee or tea a day. Do not, do not, do not even think about going on this program. Follow mine instead.

Full Version: 10-Days-10-Pounds-Off

All right. Here's the full version of my 10-Days-10-Pounds-Off Program, again with my running commentary. This is the most popular diet in my office, and the one you should go on with your doctor's permission, especially if you like grapefruit.

Breakfast

Breakfast is the same thing each day on my 10-Days-10-Pounds-Off Program.

Breakfast

1/2 Grapefruit

Coffee or Tea

If you're hungry, start your day with a 1/2 grapefruit, and as much black coffee or plain tea as you like and can get down. However, for the umpteenth time, if you're not hungry, don't eat.

No creamer or whitener or skim milk or anything in your coffee or tea, beyond Equal or SweetNLow tablets. Use Equal or SweetNLow tablets only, not the powdered Equal or SweetNLow packets in your coffee or tea. The packets contain too much hidden carbohydrate, and will throw you out of ketosis and significantly slow down your weight loss on this very rapid program. You may only use 1 packet of Equal or SweetNLow to sprinkle on your grapefruit half, not in your drinks.

If you're eating breakfast out and grapefruit isn't on the menu, you're out of luck. Carry a grapefruit with you, and pay the restaurant a plating fee to serve you half. Ask them to wrap up the other half so you can take it home with you.

If you hate grapefruit or are allergic to grapefruit, don't go on this program. Go on Dr. Nagler's 500 Diet instead (See Chapter 5).

There's no magic to the coffee or tea or Diet Coke, except that caffeinated beverages will help you feel better (giving you a caffeine-induced energy high) and burn fat faster. If you're caffeine-sensitive or caffeine doesn't make you feel good, for goodness sake don't have any. If caffeine keeps you up at night, switch to decaffeinated beverages after noon, or whatever your personal cut-off time is.

You also don't have to drink Diet Coke. My brother prefers Diet Pepsi. I don't care what you drink, as long as it's noncaloric and preferably caffeinated.

Incidentally, Diet Mountain Dew has about the highest caffeine content of any of the diet sodas.

If you're hungry and going to eat, you have to start each meal, breakfast, lunch and dinner, with your 1/2 grapefruit. The grapefruit provides bulk and fiber, satisfies your sweet cravings, and will make you feel full. If you like your grapefruit sweeter, you can put 1 packet of Equal or SweetNLow on top. You cannot have grapefruit juice. You have to start each meal with a 1/2 grapefruit if you're hungry.

There's no metabolic magic or fat-burning secret to eating grapefruit before each meal, despite the selection of grapefruit "fat burning" tablets you can buy at most health food stores. There is no magic. But from my clinical experience, eating a 1/2 grapefruit before each meal is an excellent way to satisfy your sweet cravings and make you feel full.

Drinking juice of any kind - grapefruit, orange, tomato, carrot, etc. - is completely off limits. As a matter of fact, drinking juice is one of the best ways I know to gain a whole bunch of weight in a hurry. Take grapefruit juice for example. A big glass of sweetened grapefruit juice usually contains in excess of 200 calories, and probably takes less than a minute to drink. On the other hand, one half of a very large grapefruit usually contains less than 50 calories, and takes most people 3-5 minutes to eat. Think about it. If you ate as many grapefruit halves to equal the calories in a single glass of grapefruit juice (I'm talking about 2 whole grapefruit here), it would take you close to 20 minutes, and you'd be sick to your stomach to boot.

Lunch

Lunch is the same thing each day, a safe and effective modification of the old breakfast of the Original Phony Mayo Clinic Diet. You can't, like in the old days, have up to a dozen eggs and a dozen strips of bacon. Don't even go there.

Lunch

1/2 Grapefruit

Salad

Bacos & EggBeaters (4 ounces EggBeaters with 1 tablespoon Bacos)
OR
Egg White Omelette (1 yolk and 4 whites)

Coffee or Tea

Grapefruit

If you are not hungry for lunch, for goodness sake don't eat anything. If you are hungry however, start lunch the same way you start every other meal you eat on this program. With a 1/2 grapefruit.

You may add 1 packet of Equal or SweetNLow powder on top or your 1/2 grapefruit to make it sweeter if you prefer.

After your 1/2 grapefruit, if you are satisfied and no longer hungry, stop eating. The less you eat, the more weight you will lose on this program.

If you're eating out in a restaurant, and they don't have grapefruit on the menu, you're out of luck. Bring a grapefruit with you and have them serve you half on a plate.

If you are still hungry after your 1/2 grapefruit, you can go on to the rest of the meal. Once again, if your hunger is satisfied after you have your 1/2 grapefruit, stop eating. You don't have to eat the Salad or the Bacos and EggBeaters. You'll lose weight faster if you don't eat, but (not meaning to sound like my mother-in-law) if you're hungry, go ahead and eat!

Salad

Your SALAD must consist of no more than 1 cup of a mixed salad consisting only of any combination of lettuce, cucumbers, mushrooms, onions, radishes and sprouts. NO carrots, tomatoes, or any other vegetables. No cheese or croutons.

Top your salad with up to 2 tablespoons of any low-fat, low-carbohydrate salad dressing. An acceptable low-fat, low-carbohydrate dressing means that it contains no more than 3 grams of fat and no more than 3 grams of carbohydrate per tablespoon. If a dressing contains more fat or carbohydrates per tablespoon, you can't have it.

Bacos and EggBeaters/Egg White Omelette

Lunch consists of a small container of EggBeaters (one 4-ounce carton), lightly scrambled or served as an omelette. Cook in a nonstick pan with butter-flavored PAM, Butterbuds, or your favorite fat-free butter substitute. Do not use butter, oil or margarine to prepare your eggs or egg substitute. Use all the salt, pepper, herbs and spices you like.

You may add 1 heaping tablespoon of Bacos to your scrambled EggBeaters or EggBeaters omelette, either mixed into the egg mixture before or after cooking.

Instead of EggBeaters, you may have a combination of 1 egg yolk and 4 egg whites, lightly scrambled or served as an omelette.

If you're in a restaurant, order EggBeaters and 1 strip of bacon. (Do not have more than 1 strip of bacon!) Or have them make you an omelette with 4 egg whites and 1 egg yolk, along with 1 strip of bacon if you want it. Another option is to order 4 hardboiled eggs, and eat the 4 whites and just one of the yolks. Of course, you can always leave out the yolk entirely. It is mostly fat anyway and contains about 90% of the calories of a whole egg.

Coffee or Tea

Have all the black coffee or plain tea you like, sweetened with Equal or SweetNLow tablets (no packets!) if you prefer. No creamer or whitener.

If You're Going Totally Nuts Without Dessert

If you're absolutely going out of your mind for dessert, you can have ONE of the following: 1 prepackaged, individual-sized serving of SUGARFREE Jello topped with no more than 1 tablespoon of FATFREE Cool Whip OR 1 SUGARFREE Popsicle OR 1 SUGARFREE Fudgesicle OR 1 SUGARFREE Creamsicle. You can have only 1, not 1 of each.

I don't recommend any of these desserts unless you are desperate. They will not totally kill your progress on the program. Just don't make a habit of them.

Dinner

You start dinner the same way you start any meal you plan to eat on this program.

Dinner

1/2 Grapefruit

Salad (up to 1 cup)

Vegetable (up to 1 cup)

Meat (up to 8 ounces)

Coffee or Tea

Grapefruit

You may add 1 packet of Equal or SweetNLow powder on top of your 1/2 grapefruit to make it sweeter if you prefer.

After your 1/2 grapefruit, if you are satisfied and no longer hungry, stop eating. The less you eat, the more weight you will lose on this program.

If you are still hungry after your 1/2 grapefruit, you can go on to the rest of the meal.

Salad

SALAD follows the same rules as lunch. Your SALAD must consist of no more than 1 cup of a mixed salad consisting only of any combination of the following: lettuce, cucumbers, mushrooms, onions, radishes and sprouts. NO carrots, tomatoes or other vegetables. No cheese or croutons.

Top your salad with up to 2 tablespoons (1 serving) of any low-fat, low-carbohydrate salad dressing. An acceptable low-fat, low-carbohydrate dressing means that it contains no more than 3 grams of fat and no more than 3 grams of carbohydrate per serving. If your dressing contains more fat or carbohydrate per serving, you can't have it.

Vegetable

Your VEGETABLE is limited to a 1 cup serving of 1 of the following:

asparagus, broccoli, Brussels sprouts, cauliflower, sauerkraut, spinach, string beans.

Steam or roast your vegetable without butter, margarine or oil of any kind. You may top your vegetable with butter-flavored PAM, Butterbuds, or your favorite fat-free butter substitute. Lemon juice is okay too.

Meat

Your MEAT is limited to one 4-8 ounce serving of 1 of the following:

chicken, clams, crab, fish of any kind, lobster, mussels, sardines, shrimp, tuna, turkey.

Broil, bake, roast, steam or pan fry your meat in a nonstick pan, without adding any butter, margarine or oil. Season with salt, pepper, soy sauce, ketchup, lemon juice, mustard or cocktail sauce.

Dessert

If you're absolutely still going out of your mind for dessert at dinner, you can also have the same dessert you had at lunch if you need it. You may have one prepackaged individual-sized serving of SUGARFREE Jello topped with no more than 1 tablespoon of FATFREE Cool Whip OR 1 SUGARFREE Popsicle OR 1 SUGARFREE Fudgesicle OR 1 SUGARFREE Creamsicle. Just have 1, not 1 of each.

I don't recommend making a habit of eating these desserts. But, if once in a while you just have to have something sweet after a meal, they will not totally kill your progress on the program.

2 Tips To Make It Easier

(1) Any time you think you are hungry, drink a 12-ounce glass of water. Your hunger will likely disappear. Studies show that up to 80% of the time people chose to eat, they are thirsty, not hungry.

(2) Any time you are still hungry after a glass of water, you may have a 1/2 grapefruit. This means that in addition to the three 1/2 grapefruits you eat before each meal, you can also have up to an additional three 1/2 grapefruits each day, anytime you are hungry.

In other words, you can have up to a total of three whole grapefruit a day if you are hungry. This 3 grapefruit a day total, includes your 1/2 grapefruits before meals.

It's also important to eat your 1/2 grapefruit BEFORE each meal, NOT as dessert. The 1/2 grapefruit may satisfy your hunger enough so you won't want to eat anything else, which is the whole idea in the first place.

Remember:

1 - No alcohol or coffee creamer.

2 - No lozenges, gum, mints.

3 - Only Breath Asure, Binaca spray.

4 - SweetNLow/Equal tablets only.

5 - 4 quarts (128 ounces) water.

6 - Don't eat anything else.

Tear out this page

Dr. Nagler's 10-Days 10-Pounds-Off-Program

www.dietresults.com

BREAKFAST
1/2 Grapefruit
Coffee or Tea

LUNCH
1/2 Grapefruit
Salad (1 cup)
Bacos & EggBeaters OR
1 Yolk & 4 White Omelette

DINNER
1/2 Grapefruit
Salad (1 cup)
Vegetable (1 cup)
Meat (8 ounces)

SALAD
lettuce, cucumbers,
mushrooms, onions,
radishes, sprouts - with
2 T lowfat/carb dressing

VEGETABLES
asparagus, broccoli,
Brussels sprouts, cauliflower,
mushrooms, sauerkraut,
spinach, string beans

MEAT
chicken, clams, crab, fish,
lobster, mussels, sardines,
shrimp, tuna, turkey, veal

1 - Get your doctor's approval.
2 - No alcohol or coffee creamer.
3 - 4 quarts (128 ounces) water.
4 - No breading, butter, margarine or oil.
5 - Don't eat anything else.

Tear out this page

Dr. Nagler's 10-Days 10-Pounds-Off-Program

www.dietresults.com

BREAKFAST
1/2 Grapefruit
Coffee or Tea

LUNCH
1/2 Grapefruit
Salad (1 cup)
Bacos & EggBeaters OR
1 Yolk & 4 White Omelette

DINNER
1/2 Grapefruit
Salad (1 cup)
Vegetable (1 cup)
Meat (8 ounces)

SALAD
lettuce, cucumbers,
mushrooms, onions,
radishes, sprouts - with
2 T lowfat/carb dressing

VEGETABLES
asparagus, broccoli,
Brussels sprouts, cauliflower,
mushrooms, sauerkraut,
spinach, string beans

MEAT
chicken, clams, crab, fish,
lobster, mussels, sardines,
shrimp, tuna, turkey, veal

1 - Get your doctor's approval.
2 - No alcohol or coffee creamer.
3 - 4 quarts (128 ounces) water.
4 - No breading, butter, margarine or oil.
5 - Don't eat anything else.

Tear out this page

Dr. Nagler's 10-Days
10-Pounds-Off-Program

www.dietresults.com

BREAKFAST
1/2 Grapefruit
Coffee or Tea

LUNCH
1/2 Grapefruit
Salad (1 cup)
Bacos & EggBeaters OR
1 Yolk & 4 White Omelette

DINNER
1/2 Grapefruit
Salad (1 cup)
Vegetable (1 cup)
Meat (8 ounces)

SALAD
lettuce, cucumbers,
mushrooms, onions,
radishes, sprouts - with
2 T lowfat/carb dressing

VEGETABLES
asparagus, broccoli,
Brussels sprouts, cauliflower,
mushrooms, sauerkraut,
spinach, string beans

MEAT
chicken, clams, crab, fish,
lobster, mussels, sardines,
shrimp, tuna, turkey, veal

1 - Get your doctor's approval.
2 - No alcohol or coffee creamer.
3 - 4 quarts (128 ounces) water.
4 - No breading, butter, margarine or oil.
5 - Don't eat anything else.

Chapter 5

Dr. Nagler's 500 Diet

Dr. Nagler's 500 Diet is my second most popular crash diet. It's ideal for people who eat out a lot and don't want to advertise they are on a diet, and for people who just can't hack the grapefruit on my 10-Days-10-Pounds-Off Program.

The 500 diet is very low in fat, calories and carbohydrates. If you follow the diet precisely, you can drop anywhere from a half a pound to a whole pound a day.

For those of you who want to cut to the chase, here's the quick and dirty version of Dr. Nagler's 500 Diet.

Full background and support information follows, but for those of you who want to start losing weight right now, here's the diet.

In a Nutshell: Dr. Nagler's 500 Diet

You should lose about a POUND A DAY on this program. If you're not hungry, don't eat. The less you eat, the faster you will lose weight. You will be in ketosis (See Chapter 2), so you really need to push fluid to flush out your fat, and feel at your best.

This is a very rapid weight loss program. You will experience accelerated fat burning and an increased level of energy.

You can have up to 2 MEALS A DAY, whenever you want. Each meal consists of a MEAT, VEGETABLE, FRUIT and DRINK. You don't have to eat everything on the list, but the meals have been designed to make you feel satisfied. You can eat ONE MEAL, TWO MEALS, or pick at your 1-2 MEATS, 1-2 VEGETABLES and 1-2 FRUITS throughout the day. But whether you eat or not, you must drink at least 128 ounces of noncaloric fluid a day.

Food can be eaten right out of the can, or cooked without any oil, butter, margarine or fat. That means steamed, boiled, broiled or grilled. Use fat-free mayonnaise or fat-free salad dressing, salt, pepper, relish, garlic, onion salt, and any spice (without sugar) you like. Carry a plastic fork and a can opener in your purse or briefcase, and you're in business.

Meat

Have ONE CAN (4-6 OUNCES) of one of the following meats only:

chicken in broth, clams in broth, crab in water, lobster in water, mussels in broth, sardines in mustard, shrimp in water, tuna in water, turkey in broth.

You can use fresh MEAT if you want (you'll do better with CANNED), but WEIGH EVERYTHING before cooking.

Vegetable

Have ONE 8-OUNCE WATER-PACKED CAN or 1 cup (total volume) of one of the following vegetables only:

asparagus, broccoli, Brussels sprouts, cauliflower, mushrooms, sauerkraut, spinach, string beans.

In place of the 8 ounces of canned or 1 cup fresh vegetables, you may have 1 cup total volume of a salad instead, consisting only of any combination of the following: lettuce, cucumbers, onions, mushrooms, radishes and sprouts. NO carrots, corn, tomatoes or potatoes. No other vegetables. No cheese, no croutons. Use only low-fat, low-carbohydrate dressing.

Fruit

Have ONE FRESH FRUIT (not canned, bottled or dried) from the following list only:

1 apple, 1/2 cantaloupe, 1/2 grapefruit, 12 grapes, 1 orange, 6 strawberries.

Drink

Drink water, sugar-free diet pop, coffee and tea - as much as you can and as much as you want - a minimum of 128 ounces a day.

Remember

1 - NO alcoholic beverages or coffee creamer/whitener.

2 - NO lozenges, cough drops, candy, gum (even sugarless) or breath mints.

3 - Use ONLY Breath Asure or Binaca spray for your breath.

4 - Use SweetNLow or Equal TABLETS only (NO powdered packets).

5 - You must drink at least 4 quarts (128 ounces) of water a day.

Get your personal physician's permission first, and you can start losing weight today.

Now, for those of you who want the inside scoop and glorious details, here's the full version of my 500 Diet program.

Full Version: Dr. Nagler's 500 Diet

The diet is called the 500 Diet because it is approximately a 500 calorie diet. If followed precisely, the program is designed to make you drop anywhere from one half-pound to a whole pound a day.

This diet is very low in fat, calories and carbohydrates. You will be in ketosis, an accelerated fat-burning state (See Chapter 2), two or three days into the program. As long as you keep your water or fluid intake up to about a gallon (at least 128 ounces) a day, you should feel terrific and lose weight very, very rapidly on this program.

Dr. Nagler's 500 Diet consists of 2 MEALS A DAY, eaten whenever you want.

Each meal consists of a MEAT, VEGETABLE, FRUIT and DRINK.

You must select your MEAT, VEGETABLE, FRUIT and DRINK from the permitted list of foods only. If something you want is not on the list, you CANNOT have it.

Most people skip breakfast on the program, and just have a few cups of coffee or tea and get on with their day. However, if you're hungry in the morning, have one of your meals or a piece of fruit.

You don't have to eat all the food on the list, but the meals have been designed to make you feel satisfied. You can eat ONE MEAL, TWO MEALS, or pick at your 1-2 MEATS, 1-2 VEGETABLES and 1-2 FRUITS throughout the day. But whether you eat or not, you must drink at least 128 ounces of noncaloric fluid per day.

MEAT should be eaten right out of the can, or steamed, boiled, broiled or grilled without oil, butter, margarine or fat. Remove all skin before eating. Use fat-free mayonnaise or fat-free salad dressing, salt, pepper, relish, lemon juice, garlic, onion salt, and any spice (without sugar) you like. Carry a plastic fork and a can opener in your purse or briefcase, and you're in business.

There really isn't breakfast or lunch or dinner on this program. You just eat up to two servings of the permitted MEAT, up to two servings of the permitted FRUIT, and up to two servings of the permitted VEGETABLES per day.

For example, if you are hungry when you wake up in morning, you can have an apple and a cup of coffee for breakfast. At lunch, you can have a salad with diet dressing and chicken, and for dinner you can have a piece of fish and some spinach followed by a dessert of 6 strawberries and coffee.

Drink as much water, coffee, tea,

espresso, and diet pop as you can. It is especially important to drink in the morning, even if you are not thirsty.

But remember, if you're not hungry, don't eat. You can skip an entire meal, or just eat the MEAT or FRUIT or whatever. Just don't have more than 2 servings of any category. The less you eat the faster you will lose weight.

Meat

Here's the full expanded list for you.

You may have one 4-6 ounce serving of any the following meats, up to twice a day. All canned meats must be packed in water, broth, tomato sauce or mustard, NOT oil. Once again, you cannot have canned meat in oil. The easiest and best way to follow the program is to use canned meats, because of the built-in portion control.

If you prefer, you can also prepare fresh meats. But if you do, you must weigh your portion before cooking. Better yet, have your butcher or fishmonger divide your meat or fish into individual 4-6 ounce packages. Remember the quantity of how much food you eat is very important on this quick weight loss program.

You can add 1 tablespoon of Miracle Whip Free and 1 teaspoon of pickle relish per serving to make a meat salad, if you like. You may also have salt, pepper, ketchup, mustard, cocktail sauce and lemon juice.

NO low-fat or fat-free cheese is allowed. The reason is that small quantities are not very satisfying so portion control is difficult. The same is true for luncheon meats (beef, pork or poultry). Luncheon meats are also way too high in fat and salt. Again NO low-fat cheese, NO fat-free cheese and NO luncheon meats.

Remember, you may have ONE serving, up to twice a day, of ONE of the following (4-6 ounces per serving unless otherwise indicated):

chicken
clams
cottage cheese (fat-free, 3/4 cup)
crab
EggBeaters (4 ounces)
hot dogs (2 fat-free)
lobster
mussels
sardines (packed in water, NOT oil)
shrimp
tuna (packed in water, NOT oil)
turkey
veal
yogurt (1 cup fat-free, 100 calories)

Vegetables

You may have up to a 1 cup serving of 1 of the allowed vegetables, up to twice a day.

Vegetables can be water-packed or fresh, but the amount you eat is very important on this very low-calorie, very rapid crash diet program.

You will do better if you use canned vegetables, as the amount you eat on this very rapid weight loss program is very important. You can easily get into trouble by exceeding the portion size so be careful when you do your own cooking or preparation.

If you are going to cook or prepare fresh vegetables, try to leave the grocery store with the vegetables weighed out in 8-ounce portions. This will help you stay in control on the program, as I'm sure you want to lose 5-10 pounds your first week and 5 pounds every week thereafter.

Lemon juice, soy sauce, Tobasco sauce, onion powder, garlic, dried spice, salt and pepper are all allowed. However, be careful with the stronger seasonings that leave a lingering effect in the mouth. Many are tempted to overeat to get rid of the sensation.

NO carrots, tomatoes, potatoes, peas, corn, acorn or any orange fleshed squash, parsnip or sweet potatoes. These vegetables are way too high in calories and carbohydrates for this very quick weight loss crash diet program. You can have one 8-ounce serving (1 cup) of a vegetable, up to twice a day, from the following list:

asparagus
broccoli
Brussels sprouts
cabbage
cauliflower
celery
collared greens
cucumbers
green beans
kale
lettuce
mushrooms
onions
peppers (red or green)
radishes
rutabaga
spaghetti squash
spinach
string beans
sprouts
summer squash
Swiss chard
turnips
wax beans
zucchini

Instead of the 8 ounces of canned or fresh vegetables, you may have 1 cup total volume of a salad instead, consisting only of any combination of the following: lettuce, cucumbers, onions, mushrooms, radishes and sprouts. You may top your salad with one serving (2 tablespoons) of a low-fat, low-carbohydrate dressing containing no more than 3 grams of fat and no more than 3 grams of carbohydrate per serving. NO carrots, corn, tomatoes or potatoes. No other vegetables.

Fruit

You can have one serving of fruit, up to twice a day. The fruit must be fresh, NOT dried, NOT canned, and NOT frozen. Do not go over two servings of fruit a day, and do not eat fruit that is not on this list! If you do, you will stop your weight loss from being as efficient as possible.

You will do best on the program if you stick to a 1/2 grapefruit for your fruit selection. From my clinical experience over the past twenty years, seeing thousands of weight loss patients, grapefruit works best on the 500 Diet. You'll be far less hungry if you chose a 1/2 grapefruit for each of your 2 fruit servings. If you can't hack grapefruit or it's not available, switch to one of the other fruits on the list. Strawberries are a good second choice, cantaloupe a good third.

NO pears, NO cherries, NO pineapple, NO bananas, NO peaches, NO figs, NO dried and NO canned fruit, or any fruit NOT on this list. These fruits are way too high in sugar, calories and carbohydrates for this very quick weight loss crash diet program. Fruits not on the list may stop your weight loss completely.

You may have 1 fruit, up to twice a day, from the following list:

1 apple
1/2 cantaloupe
1/2 grapefruit
12 grapes
1 orange
6 strawberries

Please

Don't eat more than 2 servings of fruit a day. Don't exceed the recommended portion size, and eat only the fruits on this list.

Drink

You have got to push fluid on this diet. Drink and whatever like a racehorse.

Drink at least 128 ounces per day of any of following:

Water
Sugar-Free Diet Pop
Coffee
Tea

Notice I have put water first on the list. There's a good reason for this. I want you to drink as much water as you can first. Then, when you're sick of water, drink the other recommended beverages. Just make sure to drink 128 ounces of noncaloric fluid a day.

Pay attention to the way you feel after drinking coffee, tea and caffeinated beverages (including Diet Coke, etc.). Caffeine triggers hunger and sweet cravings in some people. If caffeine triggers sweet cravings for you, or if you are caffeine sensitive, switch to caffeine-free Diet Coke, decaffeinated coffee, etc.

Drink as much as you can and as much as you want (of the recommended beverages only), a minimum of 128 ounces a day. Remember NO juice, NO milk, NO regular soda.

Tear out this page

Tear out this page and carry it with you in your purse or wallet. There are 3 copies of this page in the book for you.

Dr. Nagler's 500 Diet

www.dietresults.com

Eat one meal twice a day. Each meal consists of MEAT, VEGETABLE & FRUIT. If you prefer fresh food and want to cook, weigh everything before you eat it. Canned MEATS and VEGETABLES are faster and easier.

MEAT: One 4-6 ounce can of chicken, clams, crab, lobster, mussels, sardines, shrimp, tuna or turkey.

VEGETABLE: One 8 ounce water-packed can of asparagus, broccoli, Brussels sprouts, cauliflower, mushrooms, sauerkraut, spinach or string beans.

FRUIT: Fresh only (no canned). 1 apple, 1/2 cantaloupe, 12 grapes, 1/2 grapefruit, 1 orange or 6 strawberries

1 - Get your doctor's approval.
2 - No alcohol or creamers.
3 - No lozenges, gum, mints.
4 - Only Breath Asure, Binaca spray.
5 - SweetNLow/Equal tablets only.
6 - 4 quarts (128 ounces) water.
7 - Don't eat anything else.

Tear out this page

Tear out this page and carry it with you in your purse or wallet. There are 3 copies of this page in the book for you.

Dr. Nagler's 500 Diet

www.dietresults.com

Eat one meal twice a day. Each meal consists of MEAT, VEGETABLE & FRUIT. If you prefer fresh food and want to cook, weigh everything before you eat it. Canned MEATS and VEGETABLES are faster and easier.

MEAT: One 4-6 ounce can of chicken, clams, crab, lobster, mussels, sardines, shrimp, tuna or turkey.

VEGETABLE: One 8 ounce water-packed can of asparagus, broccoli, Brussels sprouts, cauliflower, mushrooms, sauerkraut, spinach or string beans.

FRUIT: Fresh only (no canned).
1 apple, 1/2 cantaloupe,
12 grapes, 1/2 grapefruit,
1 orange or 6 strawberries

1 - Get your doctor's approval.
2 - No alcohol or creamers.
3 - No lozenges, gum, mints.
4 - Only Breath Asure, Binaca spray.
5 - SweetNLow/Equal tablets only.
6 - 4 quarts (128 ounces) water.
7 - Don't eat anything else.

Tear out this page

Tear out this page and carry it with you in your purse or wallet. There are 3 copies of this page in the book for you.

Dr. Nagler's 500 Diet

www.dietresults.com

Eat one meal twice a day. Each meal consists of MEAT, VEGETABLE & FRUIT. If you prefer fresh food and want to cook, weigh everything before you eat it. Canned MEATS and VEGETABLES are faster and easier.

MEAT: One 4-6 ounce can of chicken, clams, crab, lobster, mussels, sardines, shrimp, tuna or turkey.

VEGETABLE: One 8 ounce water-packed can of asparagus, broccoli, Brussels sprouts, cauliflower, mushrooms, sauerkraut, spinach or string beans.

FRUIT: Fresh only (no canned).
1 apple, 1/2 cantaloupe,
12 grapes, 1/2 grapefruit,
1 orange or 6 strawberries

1 - Get your doctor's approval.
2 - No alcohol or creamers.
3 - No lozenges, gum, mints.
4 - Only Breath Asure, Binaca spray.
5 - SweetNLow/Equal tablets only.
6 - 4 quarts (128 ounces) water.
7 - Don't eat anything else.

Chapter 6

Other Options

If either my 10-Days-10-Pounds-Off Program or Dr. Nagler's 500 Diet is not for you, I have 3 other aggressive crash diets for you to choose from. You will still lose weight quickly.

The key is to pick one diet, and stick to it for at least 3-4 days. Then you can switch to another option, which you also must stick to for 3-4 days. You should lose 5-10 pounds your first week on all of these programs, and about 5 pounds every week thereafter.

Here are your options:

Dr. Nagler's Very Low Fat Ketogenic Diet
is my easiest program for restaurant eating.

Dr. Nagler's Ketogenic Crash
is a super speedy weight loss program if you can be good about portion control.

Dr. Nagler's Rotation
is designed for patients who like a lot of variety, and have the discipline to radically switch diet programs every 3-4 days.

Option 1: Dr. Nagler's Very Low Fat Ketogenic Diet

This is a very very low-fat, semi-free-feeding alternative for patients who do not want to go on either my 10-Days-10-Pounds-Off Program or Dr. Nagler's 500 Diet. It's almost as fast as my two main crash diet programs, and a lot easier to follow if you eat out a lot.

No one will know you are on a diet unless you tell them. You should lose about a pound a day your first week on this program, and 3-5 pounds every week thereafter.

The hardest thing about my Very Low Fat Ketogenic program is portion control. You may not have more than a normal restaurant size serving of MEAT and/or SALAD. If you go over normal restaurant size portions, you won't lose weight anywhere near as fast as you will on the 10-Days-10-Pounds-Off Diet or Dr. Nagler's 500 Diet.

<u>Normal restaurant size portions are generally 4-8 ounces for MEAT and 1-2 cups for SALAD</u>. Do not exceed these portion sizes, or you won't lose weight at a fast enough rate. You may have up to 3 servings of MEAT and up to 2 servings of SALAD per day.

If you're not hungry, don't eat. The less you eat, the faster you will lose weight.

Other Options

NO cheating. Don't eat breakfast or anything at all until you are hungry. Check your ketones with Ketostix 3 times a day (See Chapter 2).

This is a very rapid weight loss program, designed to block your appetite, accelerate fat burning, and keep you energized.

MEAT

Eat ONLY from the MEAT list below until you are in ketosis. You may have one 4-8 ounce serving of MEAT up to 3 times a day.

Lean Meat
Steak, prime rib, hamburgers, pork chops, ribs, lamb chops, veal, hot dogs. Remove all fat before cooking and eating.

Poultry
Chicken, turkey, duck, goose, game hen, ground turkey burgers, turkey hot dogs. No skin.

Fish
Salmon, tuna, swordfish, flounder, grouper, haddock, halibut, cod, scrod, orange roughy, sole, seabass, turbot, monkfish. Steamed, boiled, broiled, grilled with no butter, margarine or oil.

Other Options

Seafood
Shrimp, scallops, lobster, crab, clams, oysters. Use lemon juice, fat-free butter substitutes, cocktail sauce.

Eggs
Eggs (1 Egg Yolk and 4 Egg Whites), EggBeaters (4 ounces). Boil, poach, scramble or fry in PAM.

Eat ONLY lean meat, poultry, fish, seafood and eggs for 2-3 days.

Until you are in ketosis (See Chapter 2), you must eat only lean meat, poultry, fish, seafood and eggs. It will take 2-3 days for you to get into ketosis.

Once you are in ketosis, you can add SALAD and CHEESE (see below) to your diet, but only if you are hungry. And only if you are still hungry AFTER you have drunk at least 12 ounces of water.

Most important, remember: if you're not hungry, don't eat!

SALAD

When you are in ketosis, you are burning your own body fat. At this point, you may add one cup of salad 1 or 2 times a day, with low-fat, low-carbohydrate dressing. Use ONLY lettuce, cucumbers, onions, mushrooms, radishes and sprouts. NO other vegetables. NO carrots, NO tomatoes, NO corn, NO potatoes. You need to stay in ketosis to lose weight!

Cheese

After you are in ketosis, you may add cheese to your MEAT list. You may have up to 2 slices of low-fat cheese OR a 3/4 cup of fat-free cottage cheese, up to 3 times a day. Remember if you have 3 servings of cheese, you can't eat anything else from the MEAT list.

Drink 128 Ounces Of Water A Day

You must drink at least 128 ounces of water a day. In addition, have all the coffee, tea (no cream or creamer), club soda, diet pop and Diet Jello you want.

NO diet Popsicles, NO sugarless gum, NO breath mints and NO alcohol. Equal and SweetNLow tablets only, NO packets.

If Cheese And/Or Salad Knock You Out Of Ketosis:

If you find that adding CHEESE and/or SALAD to your diet knocks you out of ketosis, return to the original MEAT only diet (NO CHEESE, NO SALAD). And drink your water. You should be back in ketosis in 2-3 days. Then try only 1 serving of CHEESE or SALAD per day.

Cooking

Steam, boil, broil, bake, or pan fry. Trim fat and remove skin before cooking. You can use up to a teaspoon of butter, margarine or oil if you're going nuts, but control yourself. If the pan gets too dry, add a little broth or water. Season with salt, pepper, herbs, spices, cocktail sauce, fat-free mayonnaise, ketchup and mustard. Use low-fat, low-carbohydrate dressings. No breading.

Sweets and Starches

If you crave sweets or starches, and diet pop and diet Jello don't satisfy you, stop all diet pop, Diet Jello, and all poultry, eggs and cottage cheese for a few days. Your cravings should disappear.

Ketostix

Use Ketostix at least 3 times a day, to make sure you are in ketosis. You should be in small or moderate ketosis. If you are in large ketosis, you are dehydrated and need to drink more noncaloric fluids (See Chapter 2).

Exercise

Try to exercise for at least 10 minutes a day. 45 minutes is better. You must break a sweat. Try to do 3 miles on a flat treadmill, at 3-6mph, every day. Take one of my Exercise Packs before and after (page 187).

Option 2: Doctor Nagler's Ketogenic Crash

The second alternative to my 10-Days-10-Pounds-Off Program or my 500 Diet is actually the fastest of all, although a lot harder to stay on.

The diet is a bit brutal, but most of my patients regularly lose 5-10 pounds their first week, and in excess of 5 pounds a week, each and every week they are on Dr. Nagler's Ketogenic Crash, the most radical of my crash diet programs.

If you're not hungry, don't eat. The less you eat, the faster you will lose.

Make sure that you drink at least 40 ounces of water with each meal. Each meal refers to every time you eat. You need to drink a minimum of at least 128 ounces of water a day, no matter what.

Never eat more than you need to satisfy your hunger on Dr. Nagler's Ketogenic Crash. Remember, if you're not hungry, you don't have to eat! Good luck!

You may have 1 MEAT and 1 SALAD up to twice a day on this program. Once a day is better, or not at all if you're not hungry.

It is essential to limit your portion size of MEAT to 4-8 ounces per serving, no more than twice a day. Limit SALAD to 1 cup, also no more than twice a day. Here's the list for your MEAT and SALAD choices. Remember, you can have 1 MEAT and 1 SALAD, up to twice a day. And if you're not hungry, don't eat.

MEAT

Eat ONE 4-8 ounce serving, up to twice a day, of ONE of the following:

Chicken
Turkey
Tuna
Shrimp
Crab
Lobster
Egg

Chicken

Fresh or canned Chicken, broiled, baked or grilled. No skin. Make Chicken Salad with Miracle Whip Free, relish, celery and onion.

Turkey

Fresh or canned Turkey, broiled, baked or grilled. No skin. Make Turkey Salad with Miracle Whip Free, relish, celery and onion.

Other Options

Tuna
Fresh or canned Tuna, broiled, baked or grilled. Or make Tuna Salad with Miracle Whip Free, relish, lemon juice, celery and onion.

Shrimp
Fresh or canned Shrimp, broiled, baked or grilled. Or make Shrimp Salad with Miracle Whip Free, relish, lemon juice, celery and onion.

Crab
Fresh or canned Crab, broiled, baked or grilled. Or make Crab Salad with Miracle Whip Free, relish, lemon juice, celery and onion.

Lobster
Fresh or canned Lobster, broiled, baked or grilled. Or make Lobster Salad with Miracle Whip Free, relish, lemon juice, celery and onion.

Eggs
EggBeaters (4 ounces) or eggs (1 yolk and 4 whites). Use PAM. Scrambled, fried, omelette (with onions, mushrooms and green pepper), or make Egg Salad with Miracle Whip Free, relish, celery and onion.

SALAD

Limit yourself to no more than 2 cups a day of salad with a salad dressing that is low in both carbohydrates and fat. Any diet dressing you like is fine, as long as it contains no more than 3 grams of fat and no more than 3 grams of carbohydrate per serving. Only use one serving (2 tablespoons) of dressing on each of your salads.

Salad vegetables must consist ONLY of:

Lettuce
Cucumbers
Onions
Mushrooms
Radishes
Sprouts

NO carrots or tomatoes. These vegetables contain way too much sugar (there's more sugar in carrots and tomatoes than in an apple for example) and will stop your weight loss cold, on this very rapid crash diet program.

If you really want to lose 5-10 pounds a week on this diet, you're better off NOT eating any salad, if you can handle it. If you're not hungry, don't eat. The less you eat, the faster you will lose weight. Not eating makes you lose weight. Eat ONLY this list. NO cheating. Don't eat breakfast or anything at all until you are hungry. Use your Ketostix 3 times a day.

You must drink at least 12 large glasses of water (128 ounces) a day. In addition, have all the coffee, tea (no cream or creamer), club soda, diet pop and Diet Jello you want. No diet Popsicles, sugarless gum, breath mints or alcohol. Equal and SweetNLow tablets only, no packets.

This is a very, very rapid weight loss program. Make sure to drink all your water (at least 128 ounces a day; 150-200 ounces of water a day is better!) to feel at your best. The water is very important to help block your appetite, accelerate your fat burning, wash out the fat you've burned, and maintain your energy by avoiding dehydration. You literally pee away your fat, so you need to drink your water!

Cooking

Steam, boil, broil, grill, bake or pan fry. Trim fat and remove skin before cooking. You can use up to one teaspoon of butter, margarine or oil if you're going nuts, but control yourself. Spray oils like PAM are better. Using non-stick cookware makes it easier to cook with less fat. Season with salt, pepper, herbs, spices, lemon juice, cocktail sauce, fat-free mayonnaise, ketchup and mustard. Use low-fat, low-carbohydrate dressings. No breading.

Sweets and Starches

If you crave sweets or starches, and diet pop and diet Jello don't satisfy you, STOP ALL diet pop, Diet Jello, as well as all poultry and eggs for a few days. Believe it or not, your cravings should disappear.

Ketostix

Use Ketostix (See Chapter 2) at least 3 times a day, or every time you urinate, to make sure you are in ketosis. You should be in small or moderate ketosis. If you are in large ketosis, you are dehydrated and need to drink more.

Exercise

Try to exercise for at least 10 minutes a day. 45 minutes is better. You must break a sweat. Ideally you should do 3 miles on a flat treadmill, at 3-6mph, every day. Take an Exercise Pack (page 187) before and after.

Option 3: Dr. Nagler's Rotation Diet

The last alternative to my 10-Days-10-Pounds-Off Program and Dr. Nagler's 500 Diet is my Rotation Diet. This program of rotating crash diets offers the most variety and also provides quick results. If you get easily bored on diets, Dr. Nagler's Rotation may be good for you.

Pick one of the rotation diets (listed on pages 110-113), and stick to it for 3 days. Then switch to another diet on the list. After 3 days, switch again. Most of my patients lose about a pound a day the first week, and at least 5 pounds a week on this program.

If you're not hungry, don't eat. The less you eat, the faster you will lose.

Remember. You must drink at least 128 ounces of water a day on all of these diets.

You may also have one cup of salad with fat-free dressing, two times a day if you're hungry. If you don't need the salad, please don't eat it. The salad will slow down your weight loss a bit, but usually not significantly.

You may have ketchup and mustard (1 tablespoon of each per serving), and unlimited salt, pepper, herbs, spices and soy sauce.

There are 2 groups of crashes on the Rotation. The first group of crashes (Group I) are faster, because they are very ketogenic (high in protein), but they are a bit harder to stay on. You can switch back and forth between the Group I and Group II diets, but if you stick to the Rotations from Group I, you'll lose weight a little faster.

Group I Rotations

Chicken Crash
You may have up to a whole chicken a day, or one 13-ounce can of canned chicken in broth. No skin. If you want to make chicken salad, for every 6 ounces, you can use 1 tablespoon of Miracle Whip Free with a teaspoon of relish.

Tuna Torture
You may have up to one 13-ounce can of white albacore tuna (packed in water, not oil) a day. To make tuna salad, for every 6 ounces, you can use 1 tablespoon of Miracle Whip Free with 1 teaspoon of relish.

Shrimp Craze
Up to 2 pounds of shrimp, lobster or crab a day, with lemon and cocktail sauce. Add lettuce and make a salad. You may have up to 4 tablespoons of low-fat, low carbohydrate dressing per day.

Hot Dog Diet
Up to 12 Best Kosher 97% fat-free hot dogs a day, with mustard and ketchup.

Egg Crate

Up to 6 hardboiled eggs a day. Unlimited salt, ketchup and mustard.

Grapefruit, Bacos and Eggs

Up to 3 grapefruit and up to three 4-ounce cartons of EggBeaters per day. You can add 1 tablespoon of Bacos to each serving of EggBeaters if you like. Cook with PAM.

Cheese Crash

Up to 1 pound of fat-free string, shredded or cottage cheese a day, with ketchup or mustard.

Donald's Diet

Up to 3 McDonald's chicken salads a day. NO croutons and NO dressing. Unlimited Diet Pop.

Arby Diet

Up to 2 Big Montanas a day, no bun. 1 packet of ketchup or 1 packet Arby Sauce per serving. All the Diet Coke you can drink.

Burger King Kraze

Up to 3 meat-only Whoppers a day. NO bun, NO vegetables, NO mayonnaise. One packet ketchup and one packet mustard per meat patty. Diet Pop unlimited.

The Group I ROTATION diets are ketogenic, and very, very fast.

You should drop about a pound a day on them your first week, and at least 5 pounds every week.

Don't go on any of my ROTATIONS without your personal physician's approval, supervision and monitoring.

Group II Rotations

The Group II ROTATIONS are very low-fat, and extremely fast, but not quite as fast as the Group I ROTATIONS.

Yogurt Yelp

Up to 6 cups of fat-free, 100-calories-per-serving yogurt a day. Most people do best having 1-3 cups, whenever they are hungry. But no more than 6 cups per day.

Milk and Banana Blast

One banana with 8 ounces skim milk, blended together or not, up to 4 times a day.

Cereal Crash

Up to six 3/4-ounce boxes of pre-packaged cereal. You are allowed one 3/4 cup of skim milk per serving.

Apple Blitz

Up to 6 apples a day. You will get diarrhea. Do not stay on this rotation for more than 2-3 days, and stop it completely if you feel weak. This diet is great for constipation.

Cottage Cheese Crash

3/4 cup of fat-free cottage cheese, 1 fruit, 2 saltines - up to 3 times a day.

Strawberries and Cream Crash

You can have 1 cup of strawberries with 1 tablespoon of fat-free yogurt or 1 tablespoon of diet Cool Whip Free on top, up to 3 times a day.

Baked Potato Blast

You can have one baked potato, up to 6 times a day. Top your baked potatoes with ketchup or with 1 tablespoon of non-fat yogurt or 1 tablespoon of non-fat sour cream. If you want to be exceedingly lazy, make your potatoes once a day in the morning in your microwave, or get them at Wendy's.

Rice Diet

This is one of my most popular ROTATIONS. You can have 2 meals a day, LUNCH and DINNER.

LUNCH - 1 cup brown or white rice with 1 cup fresh fruit (any kind of fruit, as long as it's fresh). Some people like to chop their fruit and mix it into the rice.

DINNER - 1 cup brown or white rice with 1 cup steamed vegetable (any type of vegetable you want). Some people like to chop their vegetable and mix it into the rice.

Season with salt or soy sauce. To make it easy for yourself, cook 3 days worth of rice in advance (2 cups of cooked rice a day) in a rice cooker, in the microwave or on the stove.

I recommend using brown rice over white (or a 50-50 combination). Brown rice has a lot of fiber and is very nutritious.

Chapter 7

How To Stay On A Diet

Once again, you need to see your doctor before you start my 10-Days-10-Pounds-Off Program, Dr. Nagler's 500 Diet, or any other weight loss program. Get your personal physician's approval first. Make sure that your doctor thinks that losing weight is right and safe for you. Then start.

You already know what you should eat. You know all about calories, fat, weight loss and dieting. Knowing what to eat has nothing to do with losing weight.

You know all about the exercise you're supposed to do. You know all about the water you're supposed to drink, the fat you need to avoid, and the calories you need to reduce.

Knowing all that, why is it so hard for most people to lose weight? Why is it so hard for most people to stay on a diet long enough, and consistently enough, to lose weight and keep it off for any significant period of time?

The problem is that knowing what you need to do to lose weight isn't enough. Knowing what you need to do, is not the same thing as doing it.

The Myth Of Low Self Esteem

It's certainly not self image that keeps people fat. That's for sure. Studies show that there are just as many skinny people who hate themselves, as there are fat people who hate themselves. You could spend the next twelve years on a psychiatrist's couch learning to fall madly in love with yourself, and still be overweight.

And it's not a matter of motivation or how much you want to lose weight. I don't know anybody on the face of the earth more motivated to lose weight, than a fat person.

And don't let anyone give you a hard time about will-power. You may have the will but not the power to stay on a diet. And there is a very good reason for it. Overweight people tend to have high insulin levels which makes it very hard for them to control their appetite. So they overeat. And the more they overeat, the higher their insulin levels go. And over time, overeating effects body chemistry to such a degree that it becomes extremely difficult to make the necessary dietary changes to lose weight.

The secret to losing weight, is to eat less food than your body needs for an extended period of time. You have to find a way to effectively starve yourself. Most people find this extremely difficult especially if they have a lot of weight to lose. However, some people are brilliant at it. Take thin people, for example. Most thin adults watch their weight. They don't eat everything they want. They hold back. And when they do indulge, they don't get carried away and gain a ton of weight. They watch their intake of calories and fat, and exercise a bit more than usual, and take the extra few pounds off, before things get out of hand.

Thin people can teach you a lot about weight loss.

The Attitude Of The Thin

Eighteen years ago, I began my first weight loss study by examining the habits of naturally thin people. I interviewed over a hundred naturally thin people. I wanted to find out how they stayed thin, how they were different from the rest of the world.

I had many questions. What was it about thin people's lives, lifestyles, food choices, preferences, hair color, or whatever, that allowed them to remain in control when it came to food. I wanted to find out how thin people stayed thin, apparently without a struggle. So, I asked them.

Me: "Do you ever gain weight?"

Thin Person: "Yes."

Me: "When do you gain weight?"

Thin Person: "After Christmas, New Years, Thanksgiving, vacations, that sort of thing. I put on a few pounds any time I eat too much. If I eat too much popcorn at the movies, or eat too many sweets or go to a party and have too many drinks, I put on a little weight."

Me: "So, what do you do when you want to lose weight?"

Thin Person: "Well, I just stop eating so much."

Me: "Okay, but when you want to lose weight, what do you eat?"

Thin Person: "Nothing."

Me: "But specifically, when you want to lose weight, what exactly do you eat?"

Thin Person: "Nothing."

Me: "You don't eat anything when you want to lose weight?"

Thin Person: "Nothing in particular."

Me: "You mean you don't go on a diet to lose weight?"

Thin Person: "No, of course not. I just cut down. I stop eating so much. I don't do anything special."

Me: "But aren't you hungry?"

Thin Person: "Of course, silly. How else can you lose weight?"

So, there it was, staring me in the face. The difference between thin people and fat people was so simple, so obvious, so self evident and elementary, that I had missed it completely.

Thin people know that they have to be hungry in order to lose weight.

This is not the case for a lot of the overweight people who come to see me in my office. Most are looking for the magic "no hunger" diet. The naturally thin people in my study, on the other hand, were more realistic. They knew that they had to be hungry in order to lose weight.

So I decided to conduct another study to find out if "being hungry" was the secret to losing weight.

A Study On "Being Hungry"

In my second study, I gathered together

forty overweight people at the University of Michigan League in the spring of 1983. I told my volunteers that I was going to try to help them lose weight with a radical new approach. Simply put, my volunteers were to work on being hungry. I told them that it was okay not to eat.

They were given one single instruction: to go without eating whenever they could, for as long as they could. That was it, and I would see everyone again in two months.

The results were surprising. When we met again two months later, nobody had lost an ounce. But the shocker was that 20% percent of my volunteers had quit smoking. No kidding.

I suspected I was on to something, but I didn't know what. There's an old saying in psychiatry: "Control in any direction is control".

My instruction to "be hungry" had somehow allowed my smokers to gain enough control over themselves to kick the habit, but not enough control over their appetites to lose any weight.

The more I thought about it, it occurred to me that smoking is an easier habit to break than overeating. Smoking is something you don't have to go back to. You can give it up forever. Overeating, on the other hand, is more complicated. It is a matter of degree.

You can't give up food entirely. You need food to survive.

So what was it about my study that made it easier for some of my volunteers to quit smoking? All they were told to do was to try to be hungry. The message was loud and clear: it was okay to want food, and not eat.

And then the light-bulb flashed. Twenty percent of my volunteers made a very powerful generalization. Twenty percent discovered that it was okay to desire something and not satisfy that desire. In other words, 20% learned that it was okay to want a cigarette, and not smoke. It sort of made sense.

Even so, how was that going to help me get people to lose weight. I asked myself what was it about being hungry that was so threatening to an overweight person. What was the big deal about not eating so much? What was the cause of all the trouble? Anxiety, perhaps?

That got me thinking about flooding, a psychological technique that was used in the twenties to treat anxiety.

Flooding

The early studies on flooding started with a group of researchers who were experimenting with reptile phobias. The researchers were looking for a way to cure people of fear of snakes. They had come up with an incredible technique which yielded an astonishing result: total cure in every case. It had never been done before.

The researchers would take an individual who was afraid of snakes. They would do a brief cardiac examination to make sure that the subject had no serious heart or blood pressure problems. Then the researchers would tie the subject down to a secure chair, which was also bolted to the floor. You can guess what happened next. Exactly. The researchers dropped a very large, very slippery, very frightening snake, right in the subject's lap.

The screaming would go on anywhere from five minutes to half an hour. The subjects would sweat bullets and plead for mercy. But the torture would not let up. And then suddenly, the screaming, sweating and pleading would stop.

The reason. It certainly wasn't that each and every subject had died of fright. But rather, this brutal experiment actually worked. After a 1/2 hour of torture, each and every subject's fear of snakes had completely disappeared.

It was fascinating. Most of the subjects began to laugh. They had lost their fear completely, and the result seemed to be permanent. On a follow up study more than a year later, all subjects remained unafraid of snakes. The desensitization process, or flooding as it came to be called, never went away. All subjects tested lost their fear of snakes forever, in just one treatment.

The researchers continued their work on other problems. Total cures were reported again and again. They tried the technique on people who were afraid of heights, dangling subjects by ropes attached to the tops of tall buildings. Same results every time. When the screaming stopped, the volunteers were no longer afraid of heights.

They took subjects who were afraid of spiders, strapped them down and dropped large defanged tarantulas on them. When the shouting stopped, the subjects were cured.

Flooding swept through the psychiatric community in the late nineteen twenties, and quickly established itself as the treatment of choice to help people overcome specific fears and anxiety. And just as quickly, with the birth of anti-anxiety drugs in the early nineteen thirties, the flooding technique was soon forgotten.

Flash forward thirty years. We're in the early nineteen fifties now. Another group of researchers created a new toy, a curious finding, a brilliant idea, and a breakthrough.

The new toy was a piece of scientific equipment called the EMG or ElectroMyoGram. The EMG was a machine that was able to measure the electrical activity of muscles.

When the researchers hooked up an EMG to a subject's arm and had that person swing a tennis racket or lift a heavy object, they could record and measure the firing of certain muscles. Pretty straightforward stuff. But when the researchers had the same person just think of swinging a tennis racket or lifting a heavy object, without moving at all, the EMG still measured the very same activity in the very same muscles!

These results led to all sorts of interesting hypotheses. Advocates of the flooding technique suggested that perhaps thinking or imagining could help people to get rid of their phobias.

The flooding experts wondered what would happen if they didn't use real snakes in the flooding therapy. What would happen if they asked their subjects to imagine the snakes instead? What would happen if people who were afraid of heights, were asked to just imagine themselves dangling from the top of a tall building? What would happen to spider-phobics, if they were asked to imagine spiders crawling up and down their arms?

Would just thinking about a phobic object allow subjects to lose their fear of the real thing as well? The researchers did a number of experiments, and the answer came back a resounding "Yes!"

In experiment after experiment, the researchers demonstrated lasting phobia cures, without using actual snakes or tall buildings. Snake phobic subjects simply imagined a snake in their lap, until they felt like screaming, and the fear of snakes went away. Subjects who were afraid of heights imagined they were dangling from the top of a tall building until they experienced anxiety, and their fear of heights went away. The researchers demonstrated the same one hundred percent cure rate, using imaginary objects instead of the real thing. A new era in cognitive psychiatry was born, and the technique was called implosion therapy.

Implosion Therapy

After reviewing the results of my hunger study, I thought that perhaps implosion therapy could help my subjects "be hungry" and overcome or decondition their "not eating" anxiety.

I got my group of subjects on the University of Michigan campus back together again, and tried implosion therapy, to decondition anxiety associated with being hungry. I wanted to see if implosion might make it easier for them not to eat.

This time it worked. Seventy three percent of my subjects lost an average of more than twenty pounds, and kept it off for more than a year. You can read full results of my study in my article from Psychological Reports, which is at the end of this chapter.

I think implosion therapy works well for weight loss because most fat people experience some anxiety when they try not to eat. They really don't have an eating disorder. They have a "not eating" disorder. Fat people have no problem eating. They are overly good at it. It's why they are fat.

Here's how you can use implosion therapy to help you lose weight. You'll need a friend to read the implosion imagery to you, or a tape recorder to record the imagery yourself. You can also order the tapes I use from www.dietresults.com.

I've found it most effective to use three different types of implosion therapy to help people lose weight. The idea is to decondition your feelings about "not eating", helping you to stay focused and feeling good about yourself.

The first type is Positive Implosion Therapy which extinguishes "not eating" anxiety with relaxing, feel-good, eating imagery. The second type is Negative Implosion Therapy which extinguishes "not eating" anxiety using negative eating imagery. The third type is

Motivating Implosion Therapy which helps you to stay on your diet.

Positive Implosion is fun. It uses pleasant imagery that allows you to fantasize about eating all your favorite foods. The idea is that you'll be less tempted to cheat on your diet, because you've already satisfied your desires.

Negative Implosion is quite different, but very powerful. It uses negative imagery to get you off, and keep you off your problem foods. The technique makes foods you normally find appealing almost disgusting. Negative Implosion eliminates from your diet the foods you have no business eating in the first place. If you can't stop eating chocolate sundaes, or carrot cake, or Hershey bars, or whatever, Negative Implosion can help you.

Motivating Implosion acts like a cheerleader. It keeps you focused, dieting and feeling good about yourself as you lose weight. Motivating Implosion takes the struggle out of dieting so you won't be tempted to deviate from your weight loss program.

From my research, some people respond better to Positive Implosion, while others do better with Negative Implosion. I've found what works best for most people is to start with both the Positive and Negative Implosion imagery. Over the course of a week, you'll find yourself gravitating more toward one technique or the other. Go with the one that works best for you.

The Positive and Negative Implosion techniques used for dieting are divided into two sections: Sweet and Starch. Sweets and starches are the typical foods that cause problems for people when they go on a diet.

Let's say you tend to get in trouble with sweet foods like ice cream. Every time you try to lose weight, after a few days of successful dieting, you find yourself hitting Baskin Robbins, Dairy Queen or Haagen Dazs. Or maybe it's not ice cream that's the trouble. Perhaps it's chocolate chip cookies. Or candy.

For some of you, starches cause the most grief. It's bagels and pasta that you crave. Or maybe pizza is what makes your knees weak.

From my experience, no more than half a dozen foods cause trouble for most dieters. Make a list of your problem foods. Then pick one to start with. Once this problem food is under control, which takes about a week for most people, move on to the next troublemaker on your list. And so on.

At the end of this chapter are scripts for Positive, Negative and Motivating Implosion imageries. There are Positive and Negative Implosion imageries for the most common problem foods. Your problem food should be covered. If not, just make the appropriate substitutions in a given script. Record both the Positive and Negative Implosions for your particular problem foods. Also record the Motivating Implosion. Speak slowly and succinctly. Your implosion tape should run about 2-3 minutes.

If you don't want to record your own implosion tapes, you can choose to order them from me (www.dietresults.com, 734-422-8040 or 800-511-9769). They will be produced in recorded loops so that the tapes only have to be rewound once a week.

To keep you dieting, do one session of Positive or Negative Implosion once a day, followed by Motivating Implosion. Listen to your tapes whenever you have the time. It will take you less than five minutes. Five minutes a day isn't much to ask to keep you on track.

It doesn't matter when you do the implosion. You can listen to the tapes first thing in the morning, late at night, during your lunch break, or whenever. Just take a five minute break when you are someplace where you can close your eyes. Then follow the instructions and run through the imagery in your mind.

Don't listen to the tape while you are driving. You need to be able to give one hundred percent of your attention to the implosion to have it work for you. Besides, I don't want you driving and imploding with your eyes closed at the same time.

Within a few days, you'll get a sense of whether you respond better to Positive or Negative Implosion. Stick to the one that works best for you. After about a week, when your problem food is under control, pick another food on your list. Try both the Positive and Negative Implosion imagery for the second food item. You may find that a different implosion technique works better this time. Cravings for some foods will extinguish better with Positive Implosion, others do better with the Negative technique. In either case, it usually takes about a week to get most foods under control.

After you have completed Positive or Negative Implosion on your half dozen problem foods, just do a Motivating Implosion session, once a day.

All I'm asking for is five minutes a day to keep you on track and successfully dieting.

Motivating Implosion

Close your eyes. Now. In your mind's eye. See yourself thin. (5 second pause.) Really see yourself thin. (5 second pause.) See yourself looking exactly the way you want to look. (5 second pause.) See yourself wearing exactly what you want to wear. (5 second pause.) See yourself in the mirror, strong and slender, and exactly the way you want to be. (5 second pause.) See yourself hungry, relaxed, not eating, and in control. (5 second pause.) Now. Feel yourself thin. (5 second pause.) Feel slim. (5 second pause.) Feel what it feels like to wear exactly what you want to wear. (5 second pause). Feel what it feels like to be thin and powerful and in control. (5 second pause.) Feel exactly the way you want to feel. (5 second pause.) Feel strong and slender, feel exactly the way you want to feel. (5 second pause.) Feel yourself hungry, not eating, and in control. (5 second pause.) Now. Be thin. (5 second pause.) Really, be slim. (5 second pause.) Be exactly what you want to be. (5 second pause.) Be strong and slender, and in control. (5 second pause.) Be thin, and hungry, not eating, and in control. (5 second pause.) Be thin, and hungry, not eating, and in control. (5 second pause.) Be thin, and hungry, not eating, and in control. (5 second pause.) Now, open your eyes.

Positive Implosion 1 - Cake

Close your eyes. Now. See your favorite cake in front of you. (5 second pause.) Really see it. (5 second pause.) Look at it. (5 second pause.) Smell it. (5 second pause.) Now, take a knife and cut yourself a slice. (5 second pause.) Put the slice on a plate in front of you. (5 second pause.) See it. (5 second pause.) Really see it. (5 second pause.) Smell it. (5 second pause.) Now, take a fork and pick up a perfect mouthful. (5 second pause.) Look at it. (5 second pause.) Really see it. (5 second pause.) Now, take a bite and slowly savor it. (5 second pause). Chew and swallow. (5 second pause.) Take another bite. (5 second pause.) Enjoy it. (5 second pause.) Take another. (5 second pause.) Enjoy it. (5 second pause.) Feel completely satisfied. (5 second pause.) Feel totally satisfied. (5 second pause.) Feel completely in control. (5 second pause.) Now, open your eyes.

Positive Implosion 2 - Cookies

Close your eyes. Now. See your favorite cookie in front of you. (5 second pause.) Really see it. (5 second pause.) Look at it. (5 second pause.) Smell it. (5 second pause.) Now, break off a piece. (5 second pause.) Look at the piece in your hand. (5 second pause.) See it. (5 second pause.) Really see it. (5 second pause.) Smell it. (5 second pause.) Now, put it in your mouth. (5 second pause.) Savor it, enjoy it. (5 second pause.) Take another bite. (5 second pause.) Love it. (5 second pause.) Take another bite. (5 second pause.) Enjoy it. (5 second pause.) Feel completely satisfied. (5 second pause.) Feel totally satisfied. (5 second pause.) Feel completely in control. (5 second pause.) Now, open your eyes.

Positive Implosion 3 - Pie

Close your eyes. Now. See your favorite pie in front of you. (5 second pause.) Really see it. (5 second pause.) Look at it. (5 second pause.) Smell it. (5 second pause.) Now, take a knife and cut yourself a slice. (5 second pause.) Put the slice on a plate in front of you. (5 second pause.) See it. (5 second pause.) Really see it. (5 second pause.) Smell it. (5 second pause.) Now, take a fork and cut yourself a perfect mouthful. (5 second pause.) Look at it. (5 second pause.) Really see it. (5 second pause.) Now, take a bite and slowly savor it. (5 second pause.) Eat it, swallow. (5 second pause.) Take another bite. (5 second pause.) Enjoy it. (5 second pause.) Take another. (5 second pause.) Enjoy it. (5 second pause.) Feel completely satisfied. (5 second pause.) Feel totally satisfied. (5 second pause.) Feel completely in control. (5 second pause.) Now, open your eyes.

Positive Implosion 4 - Ice Cream

Close your eyes. Now. See your favorite ice cream in a dish in front of you. (5 second pause.) Really see it. (5 second pause.) Look at it. (5 second pause.) Smell it. (5 second pause.) Now, take a spoonful. (5 second pause.) See it. (5 second pause.) Really see it. (5 second pause.) Smell it. (5 second pause.) Look at it. (5 second pause.) Now, put the spoonful in your mouth. Savor it, eat it, enjoy it. (5 second pause.) Take another spoonful. (5 second pause.) Enjoy it. (5 second pause.) Take another spoonful. (5 second pause.) Enjoy it. (5 second pause.) Feel completely satisfied. (5 second pause.) Feel totally satisfied. (5 second pause.) Feel completely in control. (5 second pause.) Now, open your eyes.

Positive Implosion 5 - Candy

Close your eyes. Now. See your favorite candy in front of you. (5 second pause.) Really see it. (5 second pause.) Look at it. (5 second pause.) Smell it. (5 second pause.) Now, take a piece. (5 second pause.) Look at the piece in your hand. (5 second pause.) See it. (5 second pause.) Really see it. (5 second pause.) Smell it. (5 second pause.) Now, put it in your mouth. (5 second pause.) Savor it, enjoy it. (5 second pause.) Take another piece. (5 second pause.) Love it. (5 second pause.) Take another piece. (5 second pause.) Enjoy it. (5 second pause.) Feel completely satisfied. (5 second pause.) Feel totally satisfied. (5 second pause.) Feel completely in control. (5 second pause.) Now, open your eyes.

Positive Implosion 6 - Pastry

Close your eyes. Now. See your favorite pastry in front of you. (5 second pause.) Really see it. (5 second pause.) Look at it. (5 second pause.) Smell it. (5 second pause.) Take a fork and cut off a piece. (5 second pause.) Look at the piece of pastry. (5 second pause.) See it. (5 second pause.) Really see it. (5 second pause.) Smell it. (5 second pause.) Now, put it in your mouth. (5 second pause.) Savor it, enjoy it. (5 second pause.) Take another bite. (5 second pause.) Love it. (5 second pause.) Take another bite. (5 second pause.) Enjoy it. (5 second pause.) Feel completely satisfied. (5 second pause.) Feel totally satisfied. (5 second pause.) Feel completely in control. (5 second pause.) Now, open your eyes.

Positive Implosion 7 - Bread

Close your eyes. Now. See a loaf of your favorite bread in front of you. (5 second pause.) Really see it. (5 second pause.) Look at it. (5 second pause.) Smell it. (5 second pause.) Now, cut yourself a generous slice. (5 second pause.) Take the slice in your hand. Look at it. (5 second pause.) See it. (5 second pause.) Really see it. (5 second pause.) Smell it. (5 second pause.) Now, take a bite. (5 second pause.) Savor it, enjoy it. (5 second pause.) Take another bite. (5 second pause.) Love it. (5 second pause.) Take another bite. (5 second pause.) Enjoy it. (5 second pause.) Feel completely satisfied. (5 second pause.) Feel totally satisfied. (5 second pause.) Feel completely in control. (5 second pause.) Now, open your eyes.

Positive Implosion 8 - Crackers

Close your eyes. Now. See your favorite type of cracker in front of you. (5 second pause.) Really see it. (5 second pause.) Look at it. (5 second pause.) Smell it. (5 second pause.) Now, break off a piece. (5 second pause.) Look at the piece of cracker in your hand. (5 second pause.) See it. (5 second pause.) Really see it. (5 second pause.) Smell it. (5 second pause.) Now, put it in your mouth. (5 second pause.) Savor it, enjoy it. (5 second pause.) Take another bite. (5 second pause.) Love it. (5 second pause.) Enjoy it. (5 second pause.) Feel completely satisfied. (5 second pause.) Feel totally satisfied. (5 second pause.) Feel completely in control. (5 second pause.) Now, open your eyes.

Positive Implosion 9 - Chips

Close your eyes. Now. See a bowl of your favorite chips in front of you. (5 second pause.) Really see it. (5 second pause.) Look at it. (5 second pause.) Bring the bowl of chips up to your nose. Smell the chips. (5 second pause.) Now, take a chip. (5 second pause.) Look at the chip in your hand. (5 second pause.) See it. (5 second pause.) Really see it. (5 second pause.) Smell it. (5 second pause.) Now, put it in your mouth. (5 second pause.) Savor it, enjoy it. (5 second pause.) Take another chip. (5 second pause.) Love it. (5 second pause.) Take another chip. (5 second pause.) Enjoy it. (5 second pause.) Feel completely satisfied. (5 second pause.) Feel totally satisfied. (5 second pause.) Feel completely in control. (5 second pause.) Now, open your eyes.

Positive Implosion 10 - Pizza

Close your eyes. Now. See your favorite pizza in front of you. (5 second pause.) Really see it. (5 second pause.) Look at it. (5 second pause.) Smell it. (5 second pause.) Pick up a slice. (5 second pause.) See the slice. (5 second pause.) Really see it. (5 second pause.) Smell it. (5 second pause.) Now, take a bite. (5 second pause.) Savor it, enjoy it. (5 second pause.) Take another bite. (5 second pause.) Love it. (5 second pause.) Take another bite. (5 second pause.) Enjoy it. (5 second pause.) Feel completely satisfied. (5 second pause.) Feel totally satisfied. (5 second pause.) Feel completely in control. (5 second pause.) Now, open your eyes.

Positive Implosion 11 - Pasta

Close your eyes. Now. See a dish of your favorite pasta sitting in front of you. (5 second pause.) Really see it. (5 second pause.) Look at it. (5 second pause.) Smell it. (5 second pause.) Now, take a perfect forkful. (5 second pause.) See it. (5 second pause.) Really see it. (5 second pause.) Smell it. (5 second pause.) Now, put it in your mouth, slowly savor it, eat it, swallow it. (5 second pause.) Take another forkful. (5 second pause.) Enjoy it. (5 second pause.) Take another. (5 second pause.) Enjoy it. (5 second pause.) Feel completely satisfied. (5 second pause.) Feel totally satisfied. (5 second pause.) Feel completely in control. (5 second pause.) Now, open your eyes.

Positive Implosion 12 - Potatoes

Close your eyes. Now. See your favorite potato dish in front of you. (5 second pause.) Really see it. (5 second pause.) Look at it. (5 second pause.) Smell it. (5 second pause.) Now, take a perfect forkful. (5 second pause.) See it. (5 second pause.) Really see it. (5 second pause.) Smell it. (5 second pause.) Now, put it in your mouth, slowly savor it, eat it, swallow it. (5 second pause.) Take another bite. (5 second pause.) Enjoy it. (5 second pause.) Take another. (5 second pause.) Enjoy it. (5 second pause.) Feel completely satisfied. (5 second pause.) Feel totally satisfied. (5 second pause.) Feel completely in control. (5 second pause.) Now, open your eyes.

Negative Implosion 1 - Cake

Close your eyes. Now. See a slice of your favorite cake in front of you. (5 second pause.) Now, use a fork and cut a piece. Put it in your mouth and swallow it. (5 second pause.) As you go to take another bite, notice that there are worms coming out of the cake. (5 second pause.) There are worms coming out of your mouth. (5 second pause.) Look at the cake. There are worms coming out of the cake and out of your mouth. (5 second pause.) The worms are slimy and smell awful. (5 second pause.) See yourself throw up. See yourself throw up worms and vomit all over the cake. (5 second pause.) Throw out the vomit covered worm cake. Throw it out. (5 second pause.) It's gone. It's all gone. It's all gone. (5 second pause.) You don't need it anymore. (5 second pause.) You don't need it anymore. (5 second pause.) You don't need it anymore. (5 second pause.) Now, open your eyes.

Negative Implosion 2 - Cookies

Close your eyes. Now. See your favorite cookie in front of you. (5 second pause.) Now, put a piece in your mouth and swallow it. (5 second pause.) As you go to take another bite, notice that there are maggots coming out of the cookie. (5 second pause.) Maggots are coming out of your mouth. (5 second pause.) Look at the cookie. There are maggots coming out of the cookie and out of your mouth. (5 second pause.) The maggots are slimy and smell awful. (5 second pause.) See yourself throw up. See yourself throw up maggots and vomit all over the cookie. (5 second pause.) Throw out the vomit covered maggot cookie. Throw it out. (5 second pause.) It's gone. It's all gone. It's all gone. (5 second pause.) You don't need it anymore. (5 second pause.) You don't need it anymore. (5 second pause.) You don't need it anymore. (5 second pause.) Now, open your eyes.

Negative Implosion 3 - Pie

Close your eyes. Now. See a piece of your favorite pie in front of you. (5 second pause.) Now, use a fork and cut off a piece. Put it in your mouth and swallow it. (5 second pause.) As you go to take another bite, notice that there are worms coming out of the pie. (5 second pause.) Worms are coming out of your mouth. (5 second pause.) Look at the pie. There are worms coming out of the pie and out of your mouth. (5 second pause.) The worms are slimy and smell awful. (5 second pause.) See yourself throw up. See yourself throw up worms and vomit all over the pie. (5 second pause.) Throw out the vomit covered worm pie. Throw it out. (5 second pause.) It's gone. It's all gone. It's all gone. (5 second pause.) You don't need it anymore. (5 second pause.) You don't need it anymore. (5 second pause.) You don't need it anymore. (5 second pause.) Now, open your eyes.

Negative Implosion 4 - Ice Cream

Close your eyes. Now. See a dish of your favorite ice cream in front of you. (5 second pause.) Now, put a spoonful in your mouth and swallow it. (5 second pause.) As you take another spoonful, notice that there are worms coming out of the ice cream. (5 second pause.) Worms are coming out of your mouth. (5 second pause.) Look at the ice cream. There are worms coming out of the ice cream and out of your mouth. (5 second pause.) The worms are slimy and smell awful. (5 second pause.) See yourself throw up. See yourself throw up worms and vomit all over the ice cream. (5 second pause.) Throw out the vomit covered worm-infested ice cream. Throw it out. (5 second pause.) It's gone. It's all gone. It's all gone. (5 second pause.) You don't need it anymore. (5 second pause.) You don't need it anymore. (5 second pause.) You don't need it anymore. (5 second pause.) Now, open your eyes.

Negative Implosion 5 - Candy

Close your eyes. Now. See your favorite candy in front of you. (5 second pause.) Now, put a piece in your mouth and swallow it. (5 second pause.) As you go to take another bite, notice that there are maggots coming out of the candy. (5 second pause.) There are maggots coming out of your mouth. (5 second pause.) Look at the candy. There are maggots coming out of the candy and out of your mouth. (5 second pause.) The maggots are slimy and smell awful. (5 second pause.) See yourself throw up. See yourself throw up maggots and vomit all over the candy. (5 second pause.) Throw out the vomit covered maggot candy. Throw it out. (5 second pause.) It's gone. It's all gone. It's all gone. (5 second pause.) You don't need it anymore. (5 second pause.) You don't need it anymore. (5 second pause.) You don't need it anymore. (5 second pause.) Now, open your eyes.

Negative Implosion 6 - Pastry

Close your eyes. Now. See your favorite pastry in front of you. (5 second pause.) Now, put a piece in your mouth and swallow it. (5 second pause.) As you go to take another bite, notice that there are worms coming out of the pastry. (5 second pause.) There are worms coming out of your mouth. (5 second pause.) Look at the pastry. There are worms coming out of the pastry and out of your mouth. (5 second pause.) The worms are slimy and smell awful. (5 second pause.) See yourself throw up. See yourself throw up worms and vomit all over the pastry. (5 second pause.) Throw out the vomit covered worm pastry. Throw it out. (5 second pause.) It's gone. It's all gone. It's all gone. (5 second pause.) You don't need it anymore. (5 second pause.) You don't need it anymore. (5 second pause.) You don't need it anymore. (5 second pause.) Now, open your eyes.

Negative Implosion 7 - Bread

Close your eyes. Now. See a loaf of your favorite bread in front of you. (5 second pause.) Now, take a slice and put a piece in your mouth and swallow it. (5 second pause.) As you go to take another bite, notice that there are worms coming out of the bread. (5 second pause.) There are worms coming out of your mouth. (5 second pause.) Look at the bread. There are worms coming out of the bread and out of your mouth. (5 second pause.) The worms are slimy and smell awful. (5 second pause.) See yourself throw up. See yourself throw up worms and vomit all over the bread. (5 second pause.) Throw out the vomit covered worm bread. Throw it out. (5 second pause.) It's gone. It's all gone. It's all gone. (5 second pause.) You don't need it anymore. (5 second pause.) You don't need it anymore. (5 second pause.) You don't need it anymore. (5 second pause.) Now, open your eyes.

Negative Implosion 8 - Crackers

Close your eyes. Now. See a plate of your favorite crackers in front of you. (5 second pause.) Now, pick up one and take a bite. Chew and swallow. (5 second pause.) As you go to take another bite, notice that there are maggots coming out of the cracker. (5 second pause.) There are maggots coming out of your mouth. (5 second pause.) Look at the cracker. There are maggots coming out of the cracker and out of your mouth. (5 second pause.) The maggots are slimy and smell awful. (5 second pause.) See yourself throw up. See yourself throw up maggots and vomit all over the cracker. (5 second pause.) Throw out the vomit covered maggot cracker. Throw out all the crackers. (5 second pause.) They're gone. They're all gone. They're all gone. (5 second pause.) You don't need them anymore. (5 second pause.) You don't need them anymore. (5 second pause.) You don't need them anymore. (5 second pause.) Now, open your eyes.

Negative Implosion 9 - Chips

Close your eyes. Now. See a bowl of your favorite chips in front of you. (5 second pause.) Now, put a chip in your mouth, chew it and swallow it. (5 second pause.) As you go to take another one, notice that there are maggots coming out of the chips. (5 second pause.) There are maggots coming out of your mouth. (5 second pause.) Look at the chips. There are maggots coming out of the chips and out of your mouth. (5 second pause.) The maggots are slimy and smell awful. (5 second pause.) See yourself throw up. See yourself throw up maggots and vomit all over the chips. (5 second pause.) Throw out the vomit covered maggot chips. Throw them out. (5 second pause.) They're gone. They're all gone. They're all gone. (5 second pause.) You don't need them anymore. (5 second pause.) You don't need them anymore. (5 second pause.) You don't need them anymore. (5 second pause.) Now, open your eyes.

Negative Implosion 10 - Pizza

Close your eyes. Now. See your favorite type of pizza in front of you. (5 second pause.) Take a slice. (5 second pause.) Take a bite. Chew it and swallow it. (5 second pause.) As you go to take another bite, notice that there are worms coming out of the pizza. (5 second pause.) Worms are coming out of your mouth. (5 second pause.) Look at the pizza. There are worms coming out of the pizza and out of your mouth. (5 second pause.) The worms are slimy and smell awful. (5 second pause.) See yourself throw up. See yourself throw up worms and vomit all over the pizza. (5 second pause.) Throw out the vomit covered worm pizza. Throw it out. (5 second pause.) It's gone. It's all gone. It's all gone. (5 second pause.) You don't need it anymore. (5 second pause.) You don't need it anymore. (5 second pause.) You don't need it anymore. (5 second pause.) Now, open your eyes.

Negative Implosion 11 - Pasta

Close your eyes. Now. See your favorite pasta in front of you. (5 second pause.) Now, take a forkful. Put it in your mouth and swallow it. (5 second pause.) As you go to take another forkful, notice that there are worms coming out of the pasta. (5 second pause.) There are worms coming out of your mouth. (5 second pause.) Look at the pasta. There are worms coming out of the pasta and out of your mouth. (5 second pause.) The worms are slimy and smell awful. (5 second pause.) See yourself throw up. See yourself throw up worms and vomit all over the pasta. (5 second pause.) Throw out the vomit covered worm pasta. Throw it out. (5 second pause.) It's gone. It's all gone. It's all gone. (5 second pause.) You don't need it anymore. (5 second pause.) You don't need it anymore. (5 second pause.) You don't need it anymore. (5 second pause.) Now, open your eyes.

Negative Implosion 12 - Potatoes

Close your eyes. Now. See your favorite potato dish in front of you. (5 second pause.) Now, use a fork and take a bite. Chew and swallow. (5 second pause.) As you go to take another bite, notice that there are worms coming out of the potatoes. (5 second pause.) There are worms coming out of your mouth. (5 second pause.) Look at the potatoes. There are worms coming out of the potatoes and out of your mouth. (5 second pause.) The worms are slimy and smell awful. (5 second pause.) See yourself throw up. See yourself throw up worms and vomit all over the potatoes. (5 second pause.) Throw out the vomit covered worm potatoes. Throw it out. (5 second pause.) It's gone. It's all gone. It's all gone. (5 second pause.) You don't need it anymore. (5 second pause.) You don't need it anymore. (5 second pause.) You don't need it anymore. (5 second pause.) Now, open your eyes.

Implosion Study

Investigating The Impact Of Deconditioning Anxiety On Weight Loss

William Nagler, M.D.

Wayne State University
School of Medicine

Psychological Reports, 1990, Volume 66, Pages 595-600.

Summary

The effectiveness of a new model for the treatment of obesity was studied. This model assumed that obesity was not an eating disorder but a "not eating" disorder.

Obese individuals do not have a problem eating, they are overly good at it. Obese individuals have a problem not eating. They experience difficulty or anxiety when they do not eat.

The model assumed that removal of anxiety associated with "not eating" would allow obese subjects to lose weight. Wolpe and Lazarus' progressive relaxation techniques were used to decondition anxiety assumed associated with "not eating" in subjects. Inferred anxiety was deconditioned under conditions of "not eating" when imagining hunger, emotions, and cravings.

Twenty-five subjects were instructed not to follow a diet after deconditioning but to eat less and be hungry to lose weight. A control group of 10 was instructed to follow a balanced 1000-calorie diet to lose weight.

The former group lost a statistically significant amount of weight (7.5% of their body weight) over 11.9 months, while the control group subjects gained 6.5% of their weight.

The model appears to be effective for the treatment of some individuals who wish to lose weight, based upon this preliminary study. Replication with other and larger groups is essential.

Stunkard and Penick reviewed behavioral approaches to the treatment of obesity (7) and concluded that "Clinically important weight losses achieved by behavioral treatment for obesity are not well maintained."

Based upon another review of the behavioral literature, Foreyt and Frohwirth (1) have written that "the results of aversion therapy for obesity have been poor." Kaplan and Kaplan in their review (2) concluded that "Almost all conceivable psychological impulses and conflicts have been accused of causing overeating." And, Stunkard (6) has stated, "It would be difficult to find much support for the theory that neurosis was the cause of obesity." Schachter (4, 5) and colleagues reported that obese individuals tend to be less responsive to internal cues to eat than thin individuals and concluded "The single most pervasive theorizing about obesity is the assumption that overeating by the obese represents an attempt to cope with anxiety or fear or emotional disturbance of some kind. We have found no evidence to support it."

And Rodin (3), in assessing external cues to eat, concluded "The role of external responsiveness in the development of obesity has not received extensive confirmation. There are people in all weight categories who are highly responsive to external cues."

These traditional researchers view obesity as an eating disorder, a problem focused around eating behavior. But perhaps this is not the case. Empirically, obese persons have no trouble eating. They are overly good at it.

They eat more food than their bodies need. This is why they are fat. Obese individuals maintain their bulk by eating more calories than they need to burn to lose weight. Arguments of setpoint, genetics, and metabolic rate are not inconsistent with this basic point. If obese individuals are deprived of caloric intake, they lose weight. They just cannot seem to do it over the long haul.

The goal of any weight-loss program, then, must be somehow to get obese individuals to decrease their caloric intake and/or increase their activity. An attempt was made in this study to help obese individuals decrease their caloric intake by not viewing the problem as an eating disorder, but as a "not eating" disorder.

The assumption was made that the problem obese individuals have has nothing to do with eating, but they experience difficulty not eating when stimulated by a variety of internal and external cues.

If eating does not seem to be anxiety-related, perhaps "not eating" is. Perhaps obese individuals experience anxiety associated with "not eating" in response to internal and external cues. Perhaps obese persons eat to decrease their anxiety about "not eating."

If this is so, deconditioning "not-eating anxiety" associated with internal and external cues to eat, might allow obese individuals to lose weight. A preliminary experiment was designed to test this hypothesis empirically.

Method

Subjects

Subjects were selected from individuals who responded to a newspaper advertisement to participate in a weight-loss program. The study was conducted with 35 Caucasian subjects, 29 women and 6 men. Their mean age was 46.0 years, standard deviation of 12.8 years, variance 163.8 years.

All subjects in the study subjectively appeared to be working people of middle socioeconomic status with high school education, based upon attire, manners, speech patterns, and casual references to employment.

Subjects subjectively appeared to represent a small cross-section of the middle socioeconomic class community, although no measures were done to assess statistically whether or not they represented the community at large.

For the purpose of the study, subjects were divided into two groups. The study group was composed of 25 subjects, 21 women and 4 men. Their mean age was 47.0 years, standard deviation of 13.0 years, variance 169.0 years. The mean initial weight of the group was 218.2 pounds, standard deviation of 56.4 16., variance 3181.0 pounds.

The control group was composed of 10 subjects, 8 women and 2 men. Their mean age was 43.6 years, standard deviation of 12.6 years, variance 158.8 years. The mean initial weight of the group was 183.2 pounds, standard deviation of 45.5

pounds, variance 2070.2 pounds.

Subjects in the study group were followed for an average of 11.9 months, standard deviation of 1.4 months., variance 2.0 months. Those in the control group were followed for an average of 12.0 months, standard deviation of 0.0 months, range 0.0 months.

Subjects in the two groups were not controlled on other variables such as frame size, height, activity, or percent overweight, as the purpose of this study was to evaluate empirically the effectiveness of this model of treatment on a sample from the general population interested in weight loss.

All subjects were told only that they were participating in a weight-loss study. No statements were made concerning weight-loss expectations to either group. All subjects were told that they would be contacted again in one year.

Procedure

Subjects first participated in a 30-minute period of progressive relaxation, to teach them how to relax.

Subjects were then asked to close their eyes and to "see, feel, and experience" themselves not eating, while "seeing, feeling, and experiencing" being hungry.

Subjects were instructed to continue to "see, feel, and experience" themselves being hungry and not eating, until they felt anxious. Subjects were told to raise one hand when they felt they had produced a significant level of anxiety, one that they associated with wanting to eat and attempting to resist eating.

Subjects were then put through a period of progressive relaxation until they reported the anxiety was gone and they were experiencing relaxation once again.

Subjects were next instructed to "see, feel, and experience" themselves not eating, while "seeing, feeling, and experiencing" a state of emotional arousal they associated with eating. Subjects were instructed to raise one hand when they felt anxious.

Subjects were then put through a period of progressive relaxation until they reported the anxiety was gone and they were experiencing relaxation.

Subjects were finally instructed to "see, feel, and experience" themselves not eating, while "seeing, feeling, and experiencing" cravings to eat. Subjects were instructed to raise one hand when they felt anxious.

Subjects were then put through a period of progressive relaxation until they reported the anxiety was gone and they were relaxed again.

Subjects were instructed not to diet after deconditioning, but they were told that to lose weight, they needed to be hungry and to eat less food. Subjects received a postcard one month after deconditioning thanking them for their participation, and a telephone call in about a year at the end of the study to follow up on their weight.

The control group was given a copy of a balanced low-calorie diet (1000 calories per day). Subjects were told that to lose weight they needed to follow the diet. Two and a half hours explaining the diet was spent with subjects in the control group.

They were told that weight loss was based upon eating less food than their bodies needed and that they would likely have to experience hunger to lose weight. One month after being given the diet these subjects received a postcard thanking them for their participation and received a telephone call at the end of the study year to follow up on their weight.

All subjects in both the study group and the control group were not contacted for a period of one year and were left to their own devices without further reinforcement or examination during this period.

Results

Weight loss data for the groups are summarized in Tables 1 and 2. The mean weight loss of the study group over 11.9 months is statistically significant ($t_{24}=3.73$, $p=.001$). They lost an average of 7.5% of their total body weight, compared to individuals in the control group who gained 6.5% of their body weight. This mean weight gain over 12.0 months is not statistically significant ($t_9=1.05$, $p=.32$), although all but one member of the control group gained weight.

Table 1

Mean Weight (pounds) Weight Loss, and Standard Deviation

Subjects	n	Initial Weight M	SD
Study Group			
All	25	218.2	56.4
Women	21	201.5	40.8
Men	4	305.8	46.9
Control Group			
All	10	183.2	45.5
Women	8	177.6	47.8
Men	2	205.5	37.5

Subjects	n	Month 12 Weight M	SD
Study Group			
All	25	202.1	50.0
Women	21	190.9	43.2
Men	4	261.0	45.0
Control Group			
All	10	188.2	38.2
Women	8	181.6	36.4
Men	2	214.5	46.0

Subjects	n	Loss M	Loss SD
Study Group			
All	25	16.4	21.1
Women	21	11.0	11.9
Men	4	44.8	37.1
Control Group			
All	10	-12.0	9.7
Women	8	-12.8	10.4
Men	2	- 9.0	8.3

The mean weight loss of the women in the treated group is statistically significant (t20=3.91, p=.001). The mean weight gain of the control group women is not statistically significant (t7=0.68, p=.52), although all but one woman of the control group gained weight.

The mean weight loss of the treated men is not statistically significant (t3=2.41, p=.10), although all of these men lost weight. The mean weight gain of men in the control group is also not statistically significant (t1=1.50, p=.37), although all of these men gained weight.

Comparing the study and control groups, almost 75% of the treated men and women lost weight, while only 10% of untreated men and women lost weight. Only 4% of the treated group gained weight, while 90% of the untreated group reported weight gain.

Table 2

Percent of Subjects Who Lost Weight, Gained Weight, and No Change

Subject	n	Lost Wt%	Gained Wt%	No Change%
Study Group				
All	25	73.8	4.0	24.0
Women	21	68.8	4.8	28.6
Men	4	100.0	0.0	0.0
Control Group				
All	10	10.0	90.0	0.0
Women	8	12.5	87.5	0.0
Men	2	0.0	100.0	0.0

Discussion

Mean weight loss was statistically significant for treated subjects and for the women. Although all of the treated men lost weight, the loss was not statistically significant, because the sample was quite small and the variance large.

It appears that the deconditioning may be effective for creating weight loss in both men and women, although larger numbers of both men and women need to be studied for effects to be statistically significant.

A number of subjects who experienced weight loss spontaneously reported that they felt it was easier for them to experience hunger after the study. None of the untreated subjects spontaneously reported this experience.

Treated subjects also reported that they attributed their weight loss to eating less food and to being able to experience hunger more easily. It is interesting to note that three of the treated subjects who did not lose weight reported that they did not want to have to be hungry to lose weight.

Progressive relaxation to decondition inferred anxiety associated with "not eating" appears to help some individuals lose weight in this preliminary study. Further studies should now involve measures of the level of the reduction of "not-eating" anxiety following deconditioning and to assess the long-term effect on weight loss of deconditioning the "not-eating" anxiety.

The effect of periodic reinforcing by deconditioning and an assessment of the types of subjects for whom this approach may be beneficial are also worthy of investigation.

References

1. Foreyt, J., & Frohwirth, R.. Behavioral treatments of obesity. Volume 2. New York: Pergamon, 1977.

2. Kaplan, H., & Kaplan, H.. Psychosomatic concept of obesity. Journal of Nervous and Mental Disease, 1957, Volume 125, Pages 181-201.

3. Rodin, J.. The externality theory today. In A. Stunkard (Editor), Obesity. Philadelphia, PA: Saunders, 1980. Pages 226-239.

4. Schachter, S.. Some extraordinary facts about obese humans and rats. American Psychologist, 1971, Volume 26, Pages 129-144.

5. Schachter, S., Goldman, R., & Gordon, A.. Effects of fear, food deprivation, and obesity on eating. Journal of Personality and Social Psychology, 1968, Volume 10, Pages 91-97.

6. Stunkard, A.. The pain of obesity. Palo Alto, CA: Bull, 1976.

7. Stunkard, A., & Penick, S.. Behavior modification in the treatment of obesity. Archives of General Psychiatry, 1979, Volume 36, Pages 801-806.

8. Wolpe, J., & Lazarus, A. A. Behavior therapy techniques: a guide to the treatment of neuroses. London: Pergamon, 1966.

Accepted for publication March 6, 1990.

The author thanks James V. McConnell for his insight, encouragement, and assistance in the preparation of this paper. Requests for reprints should be sent to William Nagler, M.D., 16311 Middlebelt, Livonia, Michigan 48154.

Chapter 8

Now That You've Lost The Weight

Statistics will tell you that most people (98%) gain their weight back within a year. And from my experience this is true. But it doesn't have to be. There is a way to keep your weight off. And it's simple.

You Can't Go Back To Your Old Ways

You can't go back to eating the way you used to eat when you were overweight. If you do that, you're cooked. You'll gain your weight back in no time.

To keep your weight off, you have to face the hard reality that you have to watch what you eat for the rest of your life. That does not mean that you can never have a cookie, or a piece of cake, or even a slice of pizza. It's just that you can't have any of these treats very often or in large amounts.

Exercise

In addition to watching what you eat, you should also exercise on a regular basis. I recommend exercising for at least 30-45 minutes a day 3-5 times per week. Whether you choose to use the treadmill, the elliptical machine or go to an aerobics class, you should break a sweat for at least 10 minutes of your exercise routine.

It is also very important that you choose a realistic exercise program. By that I mean, one that you will actually follow. Don't choose running, if you have bad knees, and for God's sake, don't sign up for an 8:00 a.m. aerobics class, if you have trouble getting out of bed in the morning.

In the long run, exercise will help to speed up your metabolism and change your setpoint, so you can eat more without gaining weight. And as Gunther and Gurin's classic study on weight loss predicts, the 2% of people who can keep their weight off successfully exercise.

Added benefits of exercise are also improved cardiovascular health, increased sex drive and greater strength.

Dr. Nagler's No-Brainer Maintenance Program

My No-Brainer Maintenance Program gives you a foundation diet for keeping weight off. It is the diet that you should follow most of the time. Some people follow it 5 days a week and cheat a little on the weekends. Some people follow it 6 days a week. Some people follow it every day except on holidays, birthdays and vacation.

Now That You've Lost The Weight

My No-Brainer Maintenance Program will help you keep your weight off longer. If you follow it religiously, you should have no trouble keeping off every ounce you have lost for good. The program is so easy, you won't feel like you are on maintenance, and none of your friends will ever know unless you tell them.

The 16 No-Brainer Rules

1) Drink as much water as you can, at least 128 ounces a day. Have unlimited coffee, tea, diet pop, diet Jello and carbonated water.

2) When you think you are hungry, drink something first. Before a meal (basically, any time you eat) have 20 ounces of a non caloric fluid. If your hunger goes away, then don't eat. If you're still hungry 20 ounces later, fill up on vegetables.

3) If you are not hungry, don't eat. You don't have to have 3 meals a day. You can skip breakfast, lunch or dinner. Eating only twice a day may work for you. Once a day is okay too (that's my preference).

4) The less you eat, the easier it will be for you to keep your weight off. Keep your portions small.

5) Take it easy on butter, margarine and oil. Use fat-free and low-calorie salad dressing.

6) Avoid fried foods and breading.

7) Stay away from beer, wine and alcohol. These beverages stimulate appetite.

8) Hardly ever eat baked flour products. It is almost impossible to keep your weight under control if you eat bread, crackers, pizza or pasta. And forget about cookies, cakes and pies. Baked flour raises your insulin level, and makes you hungry.

9) Instead of baked flour products, have oatmeal, popcorn, brown rice, and baked potatoes. Use non-fat, low-fat, low-calorie toppings. Use ketchup, soy sauce, non-fat yogurt or butter flavored spray.

10) Limit your intake of nightshade vegetables as much as you can. Nightshade vegetables are eggplant, red/green/hot peppers, tomatoes, potatoes and zucchini. They can cause depression and sweet cravings.

11) Take it easy on fruit. It's almost impossible to keep weight off eating more than 2-3 pieces of fruit a day. Your insulin level will go way up, which will make you crave sweets and starches.

12) Avoid fruit juice. An average glass of fruit juice is extracted from approximately 4 servings of fruit. That's enough fruit for two days.

12) Limit your protein (beef, pork, poultry, eggs, fat-free cheese) to no more than a pound per day.

13) Get your protein mostly from fish (salmon, tuna, sword, etc.), seafood (shrimp, lobster, crab, etc.) and fat-free dairy products (fat-free cheese, fat-free cottage cheese, fat-free yogurt, EggBeaters and egg whites).

14) If you are allergic to or just don't like fish or shellfish, have chicken or turkey for protein instead. But it's far easier to keep your weight under control with fish and shellfish.

15) Have red meat (beef, pork, lamb) no more than twice a week. Avoid it entirely if you can.

16) Keep your intake of Equal, SweetNLow, breath mints and sugarless gum down to a dull roar. They can trigger sweet and starch cravings which tend to make you overeat.

So What About Cheating?

There will be times (given that you're human) that you will go off maintenance. You may decide to have a bagel, a glass of wine or a piece of birthday cake. Just don't let yourself get out of control. By that I mean, don't cheat very often and when you do, keep your portions small.

Not cheating very often, means different things to different people. So allow me to clarify. When you first start maintenance, be conservative. Cheat on one thing once a week. For example, have a glass of wine on the weekend. If you can handle that, cheat on two things the next week. Experiment. Everyone is different.

But a word of caution. Cheating on one thing can trigger your desire to cheat on something else. And then you lose control and gain weight. To avoid this problem, follow my No-Brainer Maintenance Program exactly as written and listen to your Motivating Implosion tape (See Chapter 7) every day.

Menu Suggestions

Breakfast

Oatmeal, sliced bananas, coffee or tea

Egg white or EggBeater omelette, coffee or tea

Bran Flakes, non-fat milk, coffee or tea

Piece of fruit, coffee or tea

Lunch

Tuna with fat-free mayonnaise, rice cracker, apple, coffee or tea

Shrimp cocktail, 1/2 cantaloupe, coffee or tea

Steamed vegetables, brown rice, coffee or tea

Egg white or EggBeater omelette with fat-free cheese and vegetables, salad with low-fat dressing, berries, coffee or tea

Dinner

Broiled fish, steamed vegetables, baked potato, coffee or tea

Vegetable soup, roast turkey, salad with low-fat dressing, berries, coffee or tea

Baked chicken, steamed vegetables, baked apple, coffee or tea

Grilled shrimp, grilled vegetables, brown or white rice, salad with low-fat dressing, coffee or tea

Chapter 9

A Visit To The Diet Doctor

What To Expect

When you first enter the reception area, you are welcomed by Sue, Shannon or Donna. They have all been on my program, and have successfully dropped quite a bit of weight. They understand what you're going through and are there to help you.

After you sign in, you will be asked to fill out a comprehensive medical history, a weight loss history, and an informed consent. This usually takes between ten to fifteen minutes.

After your writer's cramp subsides, Lisa, Kelly or Mercy (my medical assistants) will take you back into the examination area. Let's assume Lisa is the one who will be taking care of you.

Once you are in an examination room, Lisa will draw your blood for a complete blood workup to determine your blood count, serum electrolytes, liver enzymes, serum cholesterol, serum triglycerides, and blood sugar level. You'll feel just the tiniest prick in your arm as Lisa takes your blood with a pediatric 25 gauge butterfly needle. This is as close to a painless blood test as you'll ever experience.

Next comes a standard 12 lead EKG, to

assess your cardiac function and detect any abnormalities. If you've never had an EKG, don't worry. It doesn't hurt at all. Adhesive electrode pads are attached to each of your arms and legs, and another six electrodes are placed across your chest. The EKG runs for about a minute, recording the electrical activity of your heart. You won't feel a thing. The worst part is peeling off the sticky electrode pads.

After you are disconnected from the EKG, Lisa measures your blood pressure, and immediately notifies me if there are any problems. Almost once a day I have a blood pressure emergency to treat, and I usually can take care of it in the office, without having to send anyone to the hospital.

The reason I encounter this situation so often is that people with weight problems tend to have high blood pressure. It makes perfect sense given that for every pound of fat you are overweight, your heart has to pump an extra mile of blood.

But not to worry. If you are an overweight person with high blood pressure, I can help you. As you lose weight with me, your blood pressure will drop because you will be burning your body fat, taking strain off your heart. Your heart will not have to pump so much blood, so your blood pressure will go down and normalize.

Back to the program. After Lisa takes your blood pressure, it is time for you to get weighed. As you step onto the metal pad of a very high-tech electronic computerized scale, Lisa enters your sex, height, and level of athletic conditioning. I'm not kidding about your athletic conditioning. If you're a muscle-bound athlete, the scale needs to know it to take the right electronic measurements and make the correct computations.

The scale then runs an electrical current up your left leg, across your pelvic girdle, and down your right leg, measuring your body impedance. Don't worry, it doesn't hurt at all. You won't feel a thing. The computer hard disk churns for a moment as it makes various computations and calculations. It then prints out a detailed, full color, six page report, including graphs and charts, of your current health status. This report includes your weight, body fat percentage, total body water, body mass index, lean body mass, fat mass, and ideal body fat percentage.

After you are weighed, you come into my office and see me. I'm usually dressed in jeans and a T-shirt. No white coat for sure. One of the most common questions I get from a new patient is: "Are you the doctor?"

After we say hello, the first thing I want to know is what time you get up in the morning, and what time you go to sleep. I want to know about your eating habits. Do you eat 3 meals a day? Are you a snacker? What part of the day do you tend to eat the most? When do you feel the most hungry?

I ask about your level of energy. Is it usually high or low? If it's low, do you boost it with sweets or starches? Or both? If you crave both sweets and starches, I want to know what percentage of the time you crave one or the other. Is it 50% sweets and 50% starches, or 60% sweets and 40% starches, or 40% sweets and 60% starches, or whatever.

Once I have all of this important information, I customize a very specific diet program, just for you. I may recommend one of the diets in this book or my Formula Program. I also may recommend that you take diet medication or supplements to help you lose weight more easily. Some of the medications and supplements are available through my Diet-By-Mail program for times when you can't make it to see me. To help you stay motivated on your diet, I may also recommend my Implosion Tapes (See Chapter 7).

On the following pages, you can read about my Formula Program, Prescription Medication, Diet-By-Mail and Implosion Tapes. I want to give you a good idea of what to expect when you come to see me, or any other diet doctor. Remember, you need your physician's approval before starting any weight loss program.

Dr. Nagler's Formula Program

Most people lose about pound a day, or 5-10 pounds their first week on Dr. Nagler's Formula Program. Weight drops off as fast as medically possible, without hunger or cravings, or any drop in energy. This a very a popular program. It's incredibly easy and people feel terrific on it.

DR. NAGLER'S FORMULA comes in a box with a straw, ready to drink, and requires no refrigeration. Dr. Nagler's Formula Program is so easy to follow:

Drink 2 FORMULA, twice a day. I recommend 2 FORMULA for lunch and 2 FORMULA for dinner. You will feel better and you will do better on the program if you force yourself to have 4 servings of FORMULA a day, whether you feel you need it or want it.

If you are hungry have an additional 2 FORMULA A DAY for breakfast and/or an evening snack. Most people do better having 2 formula at a time, not one. No more than 8 FORMULA per day. 4 FORMULA a day is best, 6 FORMULA a day is okay, 8 FORMULA you're pushing it.

You must drink at least 128 ounces (one gallon) of fluid a day on this program, in addition to your Formula. You need this much fluid to flush out the fat you are burning, and to keep your kidneys healthy.

Drink water, diet pop, coffee or tea - as much as you can and as much as you want. Make sure you drink a minimum of 128 ounces of fluid a day, in addition to your Formula. (NO juice, milk, regular soda or creamer in your coffee or tea.)

1 - Absolutely NO alcohol. It will stop you from losing weight.

2 - NO lozenges, cough drops, candy, or breath mints.

3 - Use Breath Asure or Binaca spray for your breath.

4 - Use SweetNLow or Equal TABLETS only (NO powdered packets).

5 - Sugarless gum is okay, up to 12 sticks a day.

Prescription Medication

There are three types of prescription medication that I use in my weight loss practice: appetite suppressants, thermogenic agents and carbohydrate blocking agents. Prescription medication can help you lose weight, and keep you focused and in control.

Appetite Suppressants

Prescription appetite suppressants make you feel less hungry and can boost your energy. They can also speed up your metabolism and help you burn fat faster. You should have no side effects on prescription appetite suppressants. You should not experience the jitters, palpitations or be unable to sleep. You should feel fine on prescription appetite suppressant medication. You just won't be hungry.

Thermogenic Agents

Prescription thermogenic agents can help speed up your body's fat burning. You may feel a bit cold when you experience weight loss on thermogenic agents, but this is a normal side effect of rapid fat burning. Dress warmly during the day and use an electric blanket at night if you need to, and you should be fine.

Once again, you should not experience sleep disturbance, the jitters or palpitations on thermogenic agents. You just burn fat faster.

Carbohydrate Blocking Agents

Prescription carbohydrate blocking agents can help block your cravings for sweets, starches and alcohol. Please stay well hydrated when you take carbohydrate blocking agents (drink at least 128 ounces of water a day), or you may experience a little nausea.

If you come see me at my office, I will customize a program using one, two or all three of these types of prescription medications, based upon your metabolism, dietary habits and cravings. My goal is to create the fastest and safest weight loss medically possible.

Diet-By-Mail

If you can't come into the office, I can mail you special supplements and medication, everything you need to help you burn fat, boost your energy, and kill your cravings.

The supplements and medications available in my Diet-By-Mail program are: Diet Results tablets, Fat Packs and Diet Packs.

The Diet Results tablets are designed to help block your appetite, and the Fat

Packs are designed to help speed up fat burning without speeding you up. You should experience no palpitations or jitters. Diet Packs are designed to help specific diet problems such as binging or sweet and starch cravings.

Diet Results I, II, III & IV

Diet Results tablets are the core appetite suppressants of my Diet-By-Mail program. You take one packet of Diet Results tablets up to three times a day before meals. Four different strengths of Diet Results tablets are available, depending upon how much weight you want to lose, and how fast you want to lose it.

Fat Packs

Fat Packs are designed to help speed up your weight loss by enzymatically facilitating the break down of body fat. A nice side effect is that they can also help curb your sweet and starch cravings.

Fat Packs are a special combination of Reichi Mushroom, Siberian Ginseng, Rhodea Roseola, Artichoke and the amino acid L-Carnitine. Most Diet-By-Mail patients take a Fat Pack up to three times a day, along with their Diet Results tablets, to facilitate fat burning.

Diet Packs

Diet Packs are special prepackaged packets of tablets and capsules, designed to help specific dieting problems. For example, some Diet Packs stop binging, some kill sweet or starch cravings, some boost energy, etc. Most people take a Diet Pack one to three times a day, depending on their individual needs. Below are a list of my most popular Diet Packs:

Binge-Pack - stop night eating and binging, stabilize blood sugar

Cold-Pack - fight off colds & flu in days

Depression-Pack - lift depression, improve mood, calm anxiety

Dry-Pack - help dry hair, dry skin & nails

Energy-Pack - boost energy and increase vitality without jitters

Exercise-Pack - increase fat burning and inch loss from exercise

Hair-Pack - put luster and shine back, eliminate brittleness

Hormone-Pack - help eliminate hot flashes, night sweats, PMS

Sex-Pack - get your sex drive back, boost your sexual cravings

Sleep-Pack - stop insomnia, disturbed sleep and night eating

Starch-Pack - eliminate bread, cracker, chip and starch cravings

Sweet-Pack - block cravings for candy, ice cream and cake

Vitamin-Pack - boost immune system, fight aging

Implosion Tapes

Implosion Tapes (See Chapter 7) are available directly from my office to help you stay on my 10-Days-10-Pounds-Off-Program or Dr. Nagler's 500 Diet.

The tapes contain implosion imagery to make you lose your cravings for sweets and starches, and to keep you motivated, focused and energetic while dieting.

There are 5 six-tape sets available:

1 - Positive Implosion for Sweets

2 - Positive Implosion for Starches

3 - Negative Implosion for Sweets

4 - Negative Implosion for Starches

5 - Motivating Implosion for Dieters

All tapes are recorded continuously, so you should only have to rewind once a week.

There are also six-tape Implosion sets available to help you quit smoking and stop drinking alcohol.

Please call my office at 734.422.8040 or toll free at 800-511-9769, or log onto my website www.dietresults.com for further details, and to order your Implosion Tape sets.

About the Authors

Bill Nagler, M.D. is Detroit's diet doctor. Dr. Nagler has specialized in Weight Control Medicine for more than 20 years. That's all he does.

Dr. Nagler is a graduate of the University of Michigan, the University of California and a Harvard Fellowship. He is a Diplomate of the American Board of Bariatric (Weight Control) Medicine, and a Diplomate of the American Board of Psychiatry and Neurology.

Dr. Nagler has appeared on the Phil Donahue Show, the Joan Rivers Show, Sally Jesse Raphael, Larry King Live, CBS This Morning, Montel Williams, Jenny Jones and Jerry Springer. He is the author of THE DIRTY HALF DOZEN (Warner Books 1991) and has been featured in USA Today, Cosmopolitan and Self Magazine.

Gabrielle Nagler, M.A. is a food writer. She is a graduate of the University of Toronto and McGill University. She is the author of THERAPEUTIC CUISINE and THE CELLULITE DIET.